Sirtfood Diet

The Complete Science-Backed Cookbook for Rapid Weight Loss

Stefanie Hines

Cooking Primed Press

CONTENTS

BREAKFAST 6

Celery Juice 7

Kale & Orange Juice 8

Apple & Cucumber Juice 8

Lemony Green Juice 9

Kale Scramble 9

Buckwheat Porridge 10

Chocolate Granola 12

Blueberry Muffins 13

Chocolate Waffles 14

Moroccan Spiced Eggs 15

Chilaquiles with Gochujang 16

Twice Baked Breakfast Potatoes 18

Sirt Muesli 19

Arugula, Strawberry, & Orange Salad 20

Bell Pepper Sauté 20

Matcha Green Juice 21

Date and Walnut Porridge 22

Shakshuka 23

Exquisite Turmeric Pancakes with Lemon Yogurt Sauce 24

Sirt Chili with meat 25

Baked Potatoes with Spicy Chickpea Stew 28

Buckwheat Pasta Salad 30

Greek Salad Skewers 31

Chocolate Bark 32

Choc Chip Granola 33

Sesame Chicken Salad 34

Sirtfood Scrambled Eggs 35

Chili Artichokes 36

Not-Tuna Salad 37

Morning Egg Sandwiches 38

Quinoa Bowl 38

Sweet Oatmeal 39

Green Beans and Eggs 40

LUNCH 42

Sticky Chicken Watermelon Noodle Salad 43
Fruity Curry Chicken Salad 44
Zuppa Toscana 45
Country Chicken Breasts 46
Apples and Cabbage Mix 48
Rosemary Endives 48
Kale Sauté 49
Roasted Beets 50
Minty Tomatoes and Corn 50
Pesto Green Beans 51
Scallops and Sweet Potatoes 52
Citrus Salmon 52
Sage Carrots 54
Moong Dahl 54
Macaroni & Cheese with Broccoli 55
Glazed Tofu with Vegetables and Buckwheat 57
Tofu with Cauliflower 58
Filled Pita Pockets 59
Lima Bean Dip with Celery and Crackers 60
Spinach and Eggplant Casserole 61
Ancient Mediterranean Pizza 62
Vegetarian Ratatouille 63
Spicy Spare Ribs with Roasted Pumpkin 64
Roast Beef with Grilled Vegetables 66
Turkey meatball skewers 66
Buckwheat and nut loaf 67
Almond Butter and Alfalfa Wraps 68
Roast Chicken and Broccoli 69
Stuffed Eggplant 70
Parmesan Chicken and Kale Sauté 71
The Bell Pepper Fiesta 72
Spiced Up Pumpkin Seeds Bowls 73
Chicken & Bean Casserole 74
Mussels in Red Wine Sauce 75
 DINNER 76
Spiced Cauliflower Couscous with Chicken 77
Chicken Noodles 78
Aromatic Chicken Breast with Kale, Red Onion and Salsa 79

iv

Chicken Butternut Squash Pasta 80

Chicken Marsala 82

Chicken Skewers with Satay Sauce 83

Turkey Steak with Spicy Cauliflower Couscous 85

Turkey Apple Burgers 86

Turkey Sandwiches with Apple and Walnut Mayo..................... 87

Sautéed Turkey with Tomatoes and Cilantro.............................88

Chargrilled Beef with Red Wine Jus, Onion Rings, Garlic Kale
and Herb Roasted Potatoes..89

Orecchiette with Sausage and Chicory.. 91

Chili Con Carne..92

Lamb and Black Bean Chili 93

Tomato, Bacon and Arugula Quiche with Sweet Potato Crust 94

Beef Burritos...96

Broccoli and Beef Stir-Fry... 97

Meatballs with Eggplant..98

Slow-Cooked Lemon Chicken...99

Smothered Pork Chops and Sautéed Greens 100

Pasta with Cheesy Meat Sauce 102

Aromatic Herbed Rice..104

Herb-Crusted Roast Leg of Lamb 104

Baked Potatoes with Spicy Chickpea 105

Aromatic Chicken... 107

Buckwheat Noodles with Chicken kale & Miso Dressing.........108

Sirt Super Salad 110

Kale, Edamame and Tofu curry..110

BREAKFAST

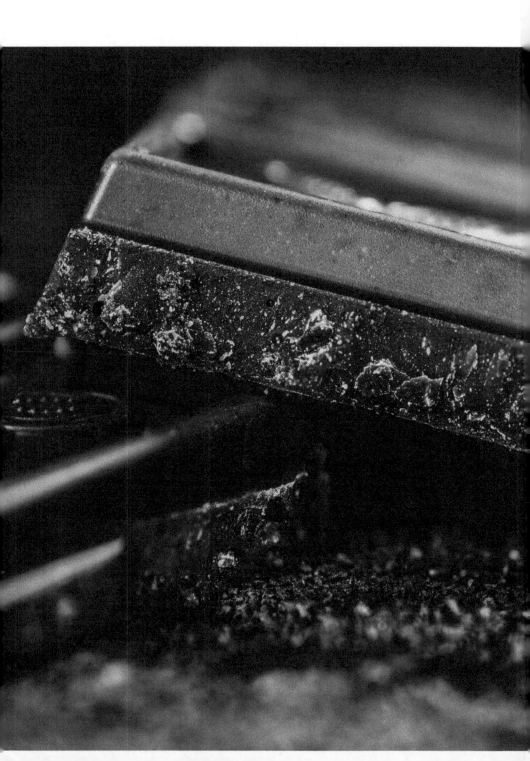

Celery Juice

Prep time: 10 minutes

Cook time: 0 minutes

Serves: 2

What you need:

•8 celery stalks with leaves

•2 tablespoons fresh ginger, peeled

•1 lemon, peeled

•½ cup filtered water

•Pinch of salt

Method:

1.Place all the ingredients in a blender and pulse until well combined.

2.Through a fine mesh strainer, strain the juice and transfer into 2 glasses.

3.Serve immediately.

Per serving: Calories 32 Fat 0.5 g Carbs 6.5 g Protein 1 g

Kale & Orange Juice

Prep time: 10 minutes

Cook time: 0 minutes

Serves: 2

What you need:

- 5 large oranges, peeled and partioned
- 2 bunches fresh kale

Method:

1. Mix ingredients into a juicer and extract the juice according to the manufacturer's method.
2. Pour into 2 glasses and serve immediately.

Per serving: Calories 315 Fat 0.6 g Carbs 75.1 g Protein 10.3 g

Apple & Cucumber Juice

Prep time: 10 minutes

Cook time: 0 minutes

Serves: 2

What you need:

•3 large apples, cored and sliced

•2 large cucumbers, sliced

•4 celery stalks

•1 (1-inch) piece fresh ginger, peeled

•1 lemon, peeled

Method:

1.Add the ingredients in a juicer and extract the juice according to the manufacturer's method.

2.Pour into 2 glasses and serve immediately.

Per serving: Calories 230 Fat 1.1 g Carbs 59.5 g Protein 3.3 g

Lemony Green Juice

Prep time: 10 minutes

Cook time: 0 minutes

Serves: 2

What you need:

•2 large green apples, cored and sliced

•4 cups fresh kale leaves

•4 tablespoons fresh parsley leaves

•1 tablespoon fresh ginger, peeled

•1 lemon, peeled

•½ cup filtered water

•Pinch of salt

Method:

1.Place all the ingredients in a blender and pulse until well combined.

2.Through a fine mesh strainer, strain the juice and transfer into 2 glasses.

3.Serve immediately.

Per serving: Calories 196 Fat 0.6 g Carbs 47.9 g Protein 5.2 g

Kale Scramble

Prep time: 10 minutes

Cook time: 6 minutes

Serves: 2

What you need:

•4 eggs

- 1/8 teaspoon ground turmeric
- Salt and ground black pepper, to taste
- 1 tablespoon water
- 2 teaspoons olive oil
- 1 cup fresh kale, tough ribs removed and chopped

Method:

1.In a bowl, add the eggs, turmeric, salt, black pepper, and water and with a whisk, beat until foamy.

2.In a wok, heat the oil over medium heat.

3.Add the egg mixture and stir to combine.

4.Immediately, reduce the heat to medium-low and cook for about 1–2 minutes, stirring frequently.

5.Stir in the kale and cook for about 3–4 minutes, stirring frequently.

6.Remove from the heat and serve immediately.

Per serving: Calories 183 Fat 13.4 g Carbs 4.3 g Protein 12.1 g

Buckwheat Porridge

Prep time: 10 minutes

Cook time: 15 minutes

Serves: 2

Ingredients

- 1 cup buckwheat, rinsed
- 1 cup unsweetened almond milk
- 1 cup water
- ½ teaspoon ground cinnamon
- ½ teaspoon vanilla extract
- 1-2 tablespoons raw honey

•¼ cup fresh blueberries

Method:

1.In a pan, add all the ingredients (except honey and blueberries) over medium-high heat and bring to a boil.

2.Now, reduce the heat to low and simmer, covered for about 10 minutes.

3.Stir in the honey and remove from the heat.

4.Set aside, covered, for about 5 minutes.

5.With a fork, fluff the mixture, and transfer into serving bowls.

6.Top with blueberries and serve.

Per serving: Calories 358 Fat 4.7 g Carbs 3.7 g Protein 12 g

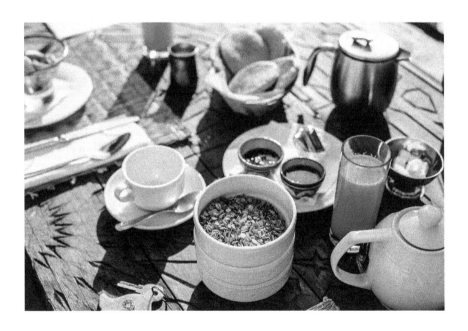

Chocolate Granola

Prep time: 10 minutes

Cook time: 38 minutes

Serves: 8

Ingredients

- ¼ cup cacao powder
- ¼ cup maple syrup
- 2 tablespoons coconut oil, melted
- ½ teaspoon vanilla extract
- 1/8 teaspoon salt
- 2 cups gluten-free rolled oats
- ¼ cup unsweetened coconut flakes
- 2 tablespoons chia seeds
- 2 tablespoons unsweetened dark chocolate, chopped finely

Method:

1. Preheat your oven to 300ºF and line a medium baking sheet with parchment paper.

2. In a medium pan, add the cacao powder, maple syrup, coconut oil, vanilla extract, and salt, and mix well.

3. Now, place pan over medium heat and cook for about 2–3 minutes, or until thick and syrupy, stirring continuously.

4. Remove from the heat and set aside.

5. In a large bowl, add the oats, coconut, and chia seeds, and mix well.

6. Add the syrup mixture and mix until well combined.

7. Transfer the granola mixture onto a prepared baking sheet and spread in an even layer.

8. Bake for about 35 minutes.

9.Remove from the oven and set aside for about 1 hour.

10. Add the chocolate pieces and stir to combine.

11.Serve immediately.

Per serving: Calories 193 Fat 9.1 g Carbs 26.1 g Protein 5 g

Blueberry Muffins

Prep time: 15 minutes

Cook time: 20 minutes

Serves: 8

Ingredients

•1 cup buckwheat flour

•¼ cup arrowroot starch

•1½ teaspoons baking powder

•¼ teaspoon sea salt

•2 eggs

•½ cup unsweetened almond milk

•2–3 tablespoons maple syrup

•2 tablespoons coconut oil, melted

•1 cup fresh blueberries

Method:

1.Preheat your oven to 350ºF and line 8 cups of a muffin tin.

2.In a bowl, place the buckwheat flour, arrowroot starch, baking powder, and salt, and mix well.

3.In a separate bowl, place the eggs, almond milk, maple syrup, and coconut oil, and beat until well combined.

4.Now, place the flour mixture and mix until just combined.

5.Gently, fold in the blueberries.

6.Transfer the mixture into prepared muffin cups evenly.

7.Bake for about 25 minutes or until a toothpick inserted in the center comes out clean.

8.Remove the muffin tins from the oven and place them on a wire rack to cool for about 10 minutes.

9.Carefully invert the muffins onto the wire rack to cool completely before serving.

Per serving: Calories 136 Fat 5.3 g Carbs 20.7 g Protein 3.5 g

Chocolate Waffles

Prep time: 15 minutes

Cook time: 24 minutes

Serves: 8

What you need:

•2 cups unsweetened almond milk

•1 tablespoon fresh lemon juice

•1 cup buckwheat flour

•½ cup cacao powder

•¼ cup flaxseed meal

•1 teaspoon baking soda

•1 teaspoon baking powder

•¼ teaspoons kosher salt

•2 large eggs

•½ cup coconut oil, melted

•¼ cup dark brown sugar

•2 teaspoons vanilla extract

•2 ounces unsweetened dark chocolate, chopped roughly

Method:

1.In a bowl, add the almond milk and lemon juice and mix well.

2.Set aside for about 10 minutes.

3.In a bowl, place buckwheat flour, cacao powder, flaxseed meal, baking soda, baking powder, and salt, and mix well.

4.In the bowl of almond milk mixture, place the eggs, coconut oil, brown sugar, and vanilla extract, and beat until smooth.

5.Now, place the flour mixture and beat until smooth.

6.Gently, fold in the chocolate pieces.

7.Preheat the waffle iron and then grease it.

8.Put the amount of the mixture into the preheated waffle iron and cook for about 3 minutes, or until golden-brown.

9.Repeat with the remaining mixture.

Per serving: Calories 295 Fat 22.1 g Carbs 1.5 g Protein 6.3 g

Moroccan Spiced Eggs

Prep time: 1-hour

Cook time: 50 minutes

Serves: 2

What you need:

•1 tsp olive oil

•One shallot, stripped and finely hacked

•One red (chime) pepper, deseeded and finely hacked

•One garlic clove, stripped and finely hacked

•One courgette (zucchini), stripped and finely hacked

•1 tbsp tomato puree (glue)

•½ tsp gentle stew powder

•¼ tsp ground cinnamon

•¼ tsp ground cumin

•½ tsp salt

- One × 400g (14oz) can hacked tomatoes
- 1 x 400g (14oz) may chickpeas in water
- a little bunch of level leaf parsley (10g (1/3oz)), cleaved
- Four medium eggs at room temperature

Method:

1.Heat the oil in a pan, include the shallot and red (ringer) pepper and fry delicately for 5 minutes. At that point include the garlic and courgette (zucchini) and cook for one more moment or two. Include the tomato puree (glue), flavors and salt and mix through.

2.Add the cleaved tomatoes and chickpeas (dousing alcohol and all) and increment the warmth to medium. With the top of the dish, stew the sauce for 30 minutes – ensure it is delicately rising all through and permit it to lessen in volume by around 33%.

3.Remove from the warmth and mix in the cleaved parsley.

4.Preheat the grill to 200C/180C fan/350F.

5.When you are prepared to cook the eggs, bring the tomato sauce up to a delicate stew and move to a little broiler confirmation dish.

6.Crack the eggs on the dish and lower them delicately into the stew. Spread with thwart and prepare in the grill for 10-15 minutes. Serve the blend in unique dishes with the eggs coasting on the top.

Per serving: Calories: 116 kcal Protein: 6.97 g Fat: 5.22 g Carbohydrates: 13.14 g

Chilaquiles with Gochujang

Prep time: 30 minutes

Cook time: 20 minutes

Serves: 2

What you need:

- One dried ancho chile
- 2 cups of water
- 1 cup squashed tomatoes
- Two cloves of garlic
- One teaspoon genuine salt
- 1/2 tablespoons gochujang
- 5 to 6 cups tortilla chips
- Three enormous eggs
- One tablespoon olive oil

Method:

1.Get the water to heat a pot. I cheated marginally and heated the water in an electric pot and emptied it into the pan. There's no sound unrivalled strategy here. Add the anchor Chile to the bubbled water and drench for 15 minutes to give it an opportunity to stout up.

2.When completed, use tongs or a spoon to extricate Chile. Make sure to spare the water for the sauce! Nonetheless, on the off chance that you incidentally dump the water, it's not the apocalypse.

3.Mix the doused Chile, 1 cup of saved high temp water, squashed tomatoes, garlic, salt and gochujang until smooth.

4.Empty sauce into a large dish and warmth over medium warmth for 4 to 5 minutes. Mood killer the heat and include the tortilla chips. Mix the chips to cover with the sauce. In a different skillet, shower a teaspoon of oil and fry an egg on top, until the whites have settled. Plate the egg and cook the remainder of the eggs. If you are phenomenal at performing various tasks, you can likely sear the eggs while you heat the red sauce. I am not precisely so capable.

5.Top the chips with the seared eggs, cotija, hacked cilantro, jalapeños, onions and avocado. Serve right away.

Per serving: Calories: 484 kcal Protein: 14.55 g Fat: 18.62 g Carbohydrates: 64.04 g

Twice Baked Breakfast Potatoes

Prep time: 1 hour 10 minutes

Cook time: 1 hour

Serves: 2

What you need:

•2 medium reddish-brown potatoes, cleaned and pricked with a fork everywhere

•2 tablespoons unsalted spread

•3 tablespoons overwhelming cream

•4 rashers cooked bacon

•4 huge eggs

•½ cup destroyed cheddar

•Daintily cut chives

•Salt and pepper to taste

Method:

1.Preheat grill to 400°F.

2.Spot potatoes straightforwardly on stove rack in the focal point of the grill and prepare for 30 to 45 min.

3.Evacuate and permit potatoes to cool for around 15 minutes.

4.Cut every potato down the middle longwise and burrow every half out, scooping the potato substance into a blending bowl.

5.Gather margarine and cream to the potato and pound into a single unit until smooth — season with salt and pepper and mix.

6.Spread a portion of the potato blend into the base of each emptied potato skin and sprinkle with one tablespoon cheddar (you may make them remain pounded potato left to snack on).

7.Add one rasher bacon to every half and top with a raw egg.

8.Spot potatoes onto a heating sheet and come back to the appliance.

9.Lower broiler temperature to 375°F and heat potatoes until egg whites simply set and yolks are as yet runny.

10. Top every potato with a sprinkle of the rest of the cheddar, season with salt and pepper and finish with cut chives.

Per serving: Calories: 647 kcal Protein: 30.46 g Fat: 55.79 g Carbohydrates: 7.45 g

Sirt Muesli

Prep time: 30 minutes

Cook time: 0 minutes

Serves: 2

What you need:

•20g buckwheat drops

•10g buckwheat puffs

•15g coconut drops or dried up coconut

•40g Medjool dates, hollowed and slashed

•15g pecans, slashed

•10g cocoa nibs

•100g strawberries, hulled and slashed

•100g plain Greek yoghurt (or vegetarian elective, for example, soya or coconut yoghurt)

Method:

1.Blend the entirety of the above fixings (forget about the strawberries and yoghurt if not serving straight away).

Per serving: Calories: 334 kcal Protein: 4.39 g Fat: 22.58 g Carbohydrates: 34.35 g

Arugula, Strawberry, & Orange Salad

Prep time: 15 minutes

Cook time: 15 minutes

Serves: 4

What you need:

Salad

• 6 cups fresh baby arugula

• 1½ cups fresh strawberries, hulled and sliced

• 2 oranges, peeled and segmented

Dressing

• 2 tablespoons fresh lemon juice

• 1 tablespoon raw honey

• 2 teaspoons extra-virgin olive oil

• 1 teaspoon Dijon mustard

• Salt and ground black pepper, to taste

Directions

1. For salad: in a salad bowl, place all ingredients and mix.

2. For dressing: place all ingredients in another bowl and beat until well combined.

3. Place dressing on top of salad and toss to coat well.

4. Serve immediately.

Per serving: Calories 107 Total Fat 2.9 g Saturated Fat 0.4 g Cholesterol 0 mg Sodium 63 mg Total Carbs 20.6 g Fiber 3.9 g Sugar 16.4 g Protein 2.1 g

Bell Pepper Sauté

Prep time: 5 minutes

Cook time: 20 minutes

Serves: 4

What you need:

- 1 red bell pepper, cut into strips
- 1 yellow bell pepper, cut into strips
- 1 green bell pepper, cut into strips
- 1 orange bell pepper, cut into strips
- 3 scallions, chopped
- 1 tablespoon olive oil
- 1 tablespoon coconut aminos
- A pinch of salt and black pepper
- 1 tablespoon parsley, chopped
- 1 tablespoon rosemary, chopped

Method:

1.Heat up a pan with the oil over medium-high heat, add the scallions and sauté for 5 minutes.

2.Add the bell peppers and the other ingredients, toss, cook over medium heat for 15 minutes more, divide between plates and serve.

Per serving: calories 120, fat 1, fiber 2, carbs 7, protein 6

Matcha Green Juice

Prep time: 10 minutes

Cook time: 0 minutes

Serves: 2

Ingredients

- 5 ounces fresh kale
- 2 ounces fresh arugula
- ¼ cup fresh parsley

- 4 celery stalks

- 1 green apple, cored and chopped

- 1 (1-inch) piece fresh ginger, peeled

- 1 lemon, peeled

- ½ teaspoon matcha green tea

Method:

1. Add ingredients in a juicer and extract the juice according to the manufacturer's method.
2. Pour into 2 glasses and serve immediately.

Per serving: Calories 113 Fat 0.6 g Carbs 26.71 g Protein 3.8 g

Date and Walnut Porridge

Prep time: 55 minutes

Cook time: 30 minutes

Serves: 2

What you need:

- 200 ml (6 ½ fl. oz.) Milk or without dairy elective

- 1 Medjool date, hacked

- 35 g (1 ¼ oz.) Buckwheat chips

- 1 tsp. Pecan spread or four cleaved pecan parts

- 50 g (1 5/8 oz.) Strawberries, hulled

Method:

1. Spot the milk and time in a dish, heat tenderly, at that point include the buckwheat chips and cook until the porridge is your ideal consistency.
2. Mix in the pecan margarine or pecans, top with the strawberries and serve.

Per serving: Calories: 66 kcal Protein: 1.08 g Fat: 1.07 g Carbohydrates: 14.56 g

Shakshuka

Prep time: 55 minutes

Cook time: 30 minutes

Serves: 2

Ingredients

•1 tsp extra virgin olive oil

•40g (1 ½ oz.) Red onion, finely hacked

•1 Garlic clove, finely hacked

•30g (1 oz.) Celery, finely hacked

•1 Bird's eye stew, finely hacked

•1 tsp ground cumin

•1 tsp ground turmeric

•1 tsp Paprika

•400g (14 oz.) Tinned hacked tomatoes

•30g (1 oz.) Kale stems expelled and generally hacked

•1 tbsp Chopped parsley

•2 Medium eggs

Method:

1. Heat a little, profound sided skillet over medium-low warmth. Include the oil and fry the onion, garlic, celery, stew and flavors for 1–2 minutes.
2. Add the tomatoes, at that point, leave the sauce to stew tenderly for 20 minutes, mixing incidentally.
3. Add the kale and cook for a more 5 minutes. If you realize the sauce is getting excessively thick, just include a little water. At the point when your sauce has a pleasant creamy consistency, mix in the parsley.
4. Make two small wells in the sauce and split each egg into them. Decrease the warmth to its most minimal

setting and spread the container with a cover or foil. Put the eggs to cook for 10–12 minutes, so, all in all, the whites ought to be firm while the yolks are as yet runny. Cook a further 3–4 minutes if you lean toward the eggs to be firm. Serve promptly – in a perfect world directly from the skillet.

Per serving: Calories: 135 kcal Protein: 9.41 g Fat: 6.16 g Carbohydrates: 12.65 g

Exquisite Turmeric Pancakes with Lemon Yogurt Sauce

Prep time: 45 minutes

Cook time: 15 minutes

Serves: 8

What you need:

For the Yogurt Sauce

•1 cup plain Greek yogurt

•1 garlic clove, minced

•1 to 2 tablespoons lemon juice (from 1 lemon), to taste

•¼ teaspoon ground turmeric

•10 crisp mint leaves, minced

•2 teaspoons lemon zest (from 1 lemon)

For the Pancakes

•2 teaspoons ground turmeric

•1½ teaspoons ground cumin

•1 teaspoon salt

•1 teaspoon ground coriander

•½ teaspoon garlic powder

•½ teaspoon naturally ground dark pepper

- 1 head broccoli, cut into florets
- 3 enormous eggs, gently beaten
- 2 tablespoons plain unsweetened almond milk
- 1 cup almond flour
- 4 teaspoons coconut oil

Method:

1. Make the yogurt sauce. Join the yogurt, garlic, lemon juice, turmeric, mint and pizzazz in a bowl. Taste and enjoy with more lemon juice, if possible. Keep in a safe spot or freeze until prepared to serve.
2. Make the flapjacks. In a little bowl, join the turmeric, cumin, salt, coriander, garlic and pepper.
3. Spot the broccoli in a nourishment processor, and heartbeat until the florets are separated into little pieces. Move the broccoli to an enormous bowl and include the eggs, almond milk, and almond flour. Mix in the flavor blend and consolidate well.
4. Heat 1 teaspoon of the coconut oil in a nonstick dish over medium-low heat. Empty ¼ cup player into the skillet. Cook the hotcake until little air pockets start to show up superficially and the base is brilliant darker, 2 to 3 minutes. Flip over and cook the hotcake for 2 to 3 minutes more. To keep warm, move the cooked hotcakes to a stove safe dish and spot in a 200°F oven.
5. Keep making the staying 3 hotcakes, utilizing the rest of the oil and player.

Per serving: Calories: 262 kcal Protein: 11.68 g Fat: 19.28 g Carbohydrates: 12.06 g

Sirt Chili with meat

Prep time: 1 hour 20 minutes

Cook time: 1 hour 3 minutes

Serves: 4

Ingredients

- 1 red onion, finely cleaved
- 3 garlic cloves, finely cleaved
- 2 Bird's Eye chili, finely hacked
- 1 tbsp additional virgin olive oil
- 1 tbsp ground cumin
- 1 tbsp ground turmeric
- 400g (14 oz.) lean minced hamburger (5 percent fat)
- 150ml (5 fl. oz.) red wine
- 1 red pepper, cored, seeds evacuated and cut into reduced down pieces
- 2 x 400g (14 oz.) tins cleaved tomatoes
- 1 tbsp tomato purée
- 1 tbsp cocoa powder
- 150g (5 5/8 oz.) tinned kidney beans
- 300ml (10 fl. oz.) hamburger stock
- 5g (3/16oz.) coriander, cleaved
- 5g (3/16oz.) parsley, cleaved
- 160g (6 oz.) buckwheat

Directions

In a meal, fry the onion, garlic and bean stew in the oil over a medium heat for 2-3 minutes, at that point include the flavors and cook for a moment.

Include the minced hamburger and dark colored over a high heat. Include the red wine and permit it to rise to decrease it considerably.

Include the red pepper, tomatoes, tomato purée, cocoa, kidney beans and stock and leave to stew for 60 minutes.

You may need to add a little water to accomplish a thick, clingy consistency. Just before serving, mix in the hacked herbs.

In the interim, cook the buckwheat as indicated by the bundle guidelines and present with the stew.

Per serving: Calories: 346 kcal Protein: 14.11 g Fat: 11.37 g Carbohydrates: 49.25 g

Chickpea, Quinoa and Turmeric Curry Recipe

Prep time: 1 hour 10 minutes

Cook time: 1 hour

Serves: 6

Ingredients

•500g (17 ½ oz.) new potatoes, split

•3 garlic cloves, squashed

•3 teaspoons ground turmeric

•1 teaspoon ground coriander

•1 teaspoon stew drops or powder

•1 teaspoon ground ginger

•400g (14 oz.) container of coconut milk

•1 tbsp tomato purée

•400g (14 oz.) container of slashed tomatoes

•Salt and pepper

•180g (6 ¼ oz.) quinoa

•400g (14 oz.) container of chickpeas, depleted and flushed

•150g (6 oz.) spinach

Method:

1. Spot the potatoes in a dish of cold water and bring to the boil, at that point let them cook for around 25

minutes until you can undoubtedly stick a blade through them. Channel them well.

2. Spot the potatoes in an enormous skillet and include the garlic, turmeric, coriander, bean stew, ginger, coconut milk, tomato purée and tomatoes. Bring to the boil, season with salt and pepper, at that point include the quinoa with a cup of simply boil water (300ml - 10 fl. oz.).

3. Diminish the heat to a stew, place the top on and permit to cook. Throughout the following 30 minutes, blending at regular intervals or so to ensure nothing adheres to the base. (This is a significant long Cook time, yet this is to what extent quinoa takes to cook in every one of these What you need: as opposed to simply in water.) Halfway through cooking, include the chickpeas. When there are only 5 minutes left, include the spinach and mix it in until it withers. Once the quinoa has cooked and is cushioned, not crunchy, it's prepared.

4. On the off chance that you like a touch of heat, add a cut red bean stew to the cooking curry simultaneously as different flavors.

Per serving: Calories: 609 kcal Protein: 23.04 g Fat: 22.15 g Carbohydrates: 85.27 g

Baked Potatoes with Spicy Chickpea Stew

Prep time: 10 minutes

Cook time: 1 hour

Serves: 4-6

Ingredients

•4-6 baking potatoes, pricked all over

•2 tablespoons olive oil

•2 red onions, finely chopped

- 4 cloves garlic, grated or crushed
- 2cm (0,8 inch) ginger, grated
- ½ -2 teaspoons chilli flakes (depending on how hot you like things)
- 2 tablespoons cumin seeds
- 2 tablespoons turmeric
- Splash of water
- 2 x 400g (14 oz.) tins chopped tomatoes
- 2 tablespoons unsweetened cocoa powder (or cacao)
- 2 x 400g (14 oz.) tins chickpeas (or kidney beans if you prefer) including the chickpea water DON'T DRAIN!!
- 2 yellow peppers (or whatever color you prefer!), chopped into bite size pieces
- 2 tablespoons parsley plus extra for garnish
- Salt and pepper to taste (optional)
- Side salad

Method:

1. Preheat the oven to 200C (390°F).
2. Meanwhile prepare all the other ingredients.
3. When the oven is hot enough, then put your baking potatoes in the oven.
4. Cook for 1 hour. Once the potatoes are in the oven, then place the olive oil and chopped red onion in a large wide saucepan.
5. Cook it gently, with the lid on for 5 minutes.
6. Continue cooking until the onions are soft but not brown.
7. Remove the lid. Add the garlic, ginger, cumin and chili.
8. Now cook for a minute on low heat.
9. Then add the turmeric and a tiny splash of water and cook for one minute.

10. Take care that pan does get too dry. Now add in the tomatoes, cocoa powder (or cacao), chickpeas (also include the chickpea water). Also, add yellow pepper and bring to boil.
11. Simmer on a low heat for about 45 minutes. Hence the sauce is thick (but don't let it burn!).
12. The stew should be cooked roughly at the same time as the potatoes.
13. Finally, stir in the two tablespoons of parsley, and some salt and pepper if you wish.
14. Finally, serve the stew on top of the baked potatoes.

Per serving: Calories: 322 kcal Protein: 8.08 g Fat: 5.97 g Carbohydrates: 61.85 g

Buckwheat Pasta Salad

Prep time: 30 minutes

Cook time: 0 minutes

Serves 1

Ingredients

• 50g (1 5/8 oz.) buckwheat pasta

• Large handful of rockets

• A small handful of basil leaves

• 8 cherry tomatoes, halved

• ½ avocado, diced

• 10 olives

• 1 tbsp extra virgin olive oil

• 20g (¾ oz.) pine nuts

Method:

1. Combine all the ingredients. Don't include the pine nuts. Arrange on a plate. Scatter the pine nuts over the top.

Per serving: Calories: 440 kcal Protein: 6.82 g Fat: 39.33 g Carbohydrates: 22.48 g

Greek Salad Skewers

Prep time: 45 minutes

Cook time: 10 minutes

Serves: 2

What you need:

•2 wooden skewers, soaked in water for 30 minutes before use

•8 large black olives

•8 cherry tomatoes

•1 yellow pepper, cut into eight squares

•½ red onion, chopped in half and separated into eight pieces

•100g (3 ½ oz.) (about 10cm (4 inch)) cucumber, cut into four slices and halved

•100g (3 ½ oz.) feta, cut into 8 cubes

For the dressing

•1 tbsp extra virgin olive oil

•Juice of ½ lemon

•1 tsp balsamic vinegar

•½ clove garlic, peeled and crushed

•Few leaves of basil, finely chopped (or ½ tsp dried mixed herbs to replace basil and oregano)

•Few leaves oregano (finely chopped)

•Generous seasoning of salt and ground black pepper

Method:

First of all, thread each skewer with the salad ingredients in the following order: - Olive, Tomato, Yellow pepper, Red onion,

Cucumber, Feta, Tomato, Olive, Yellow pepper, Red onion, Cucumber, and Feta.

Now place all the dressing ingredients in a small bowl. Mix together and pour over the skewers.

Per serving: Calories: 287 kcal Protein: 19.5 g Fat: 17.45 g Carbohydrates: 14.84 g

Chocolate Bark

Prep time: 30 minutes

Cook time: 3 hours

Serves: 2

What you need:

•1 thin peel orange

•¾ cup pistachio nuts, roasted, chilled and chopped into large pieces

•¼ cup hazelnuts, toasted, chilled, peeled and chopped into large pieces

•¼ cup pumpkin seeds, toasted and chilled

•1 tablespoon chia seeds

•1 tablespoon sesame seeds, toasted and cooled

•1 teaspoon grated orange peel

•1 cardamom pod, finely crushed and sieved

•12 ounces (340 g) tempered, dairy-free dark chocolate (85% cocoa content)

•2 teaspoons flaky sea salt

•Candy or candy thermometer

Method:

2. Preheat the oven to 100-150°F (66 ° C). Line a baking sheet with parchment paper.

3. Finely slice the orange crosswise and place it on the prepared baking sheet. Bake for 2 to 3 hours until dry but slightly sticky. Remove it from the oven and let it cool.
4. When they cool enough to handle them, cut the orange slices into fragments; set them aside.
5. In a large bowl, mix the nuts, seeds, and grated orange peel until completely combined. Place the mixture in a single layer on a baking sheet lined with kitchen parchment. Set it aside.
6. Melt the chocolate in a water bath until it reaches 88 to 90°F (32 to 33°C) and pours it over the nut mixture to cover it completely.
7. When the chocolate is semi-cold but still sticky, sprinkle the surface with sea salt and pieces of orange.
8. Place the mixture in a cold area of your kitchen or refrigerate until the crust cools completely, and cut it into bite-sized pieces.

Per serving: Protein: 20.7 g Calories: 523 kcal Fat: 40.76 g Carbohydrates: 26.65 g

Choc Chip Granola

Prep time: 55 minutes

Cook time: 20 minutes

Serves: 2

What you need:

•200g (7 oz.) large oat flakes

•Roughly 50 g (1 5/8 oz.) pecan nuts chopped

•3 tablespoons of light olive oil

•20g (¾ oz.) butter

•1 tablespoon of dark brown sugar

•2 tbsp rice syrup

•60 g (2 oz.) of good quality (70%) dark chocolate shavings

Method:

1. Oven preheats to 160°C (320°F) (140 ° C fan / Gas 3). Line a large baking tray with a sheet of silicone or parchment for baking.
2. In a large bowl, combine the oats and pecans. Heat the olive oil, butter, brown sugar, and rice malt syrup gently in a small non-stick pan until the butter has melted, and the sugar and syrup dissolve. Do not let boil. Pour the syrup over the oats and stir thoroughly until fully covered with the oats.
3. Spread the granola over the baking tray and spread right into the corners. Leave the mixture clumps with spacing, instead of even spreading. Bake for 20 minutes in the oven until golden brown is just tinged at the edges. Remove from the oven, and leave completely to cool on the tray.
4. When cold, split with your fingers any larger lumps on the tray and then mix them in the chocolate chips. Put the granola in an airtight tub or jar, or pour it. The granola is to last for at least 2 weeks.

Per serving: Calories: 914 kcal Protein: 40.19 g Fat: 63.05 g Carbohydrates: 88.74 g

Sesame Chicken Salad

Prep time: 30 minutes

Cook time: 12 minutes

Serves: 2

Ingredients

•1 tablespoon of sesame seeds

•1 cucumber, peeled, deseeded and sliced

•100g (3 ½ oz.) baby kale, roughly chopped

•60g pak choi, finely shredded

- ½ red onion, finely sliced
- 20g (¾ oz.) parsley, chopped
- 150g (5 ¼ oz.) cooked chicken, shredded

For the dressing:

- 1 tablespoon of extra virgin olive oil
- 1 teaspoon of sesame oil
- 1 lime
- 1 teaspoon of clear honey
- 2 teaspoons of soy sauce

Method:

1. In a dry frying pan, put the sesame seeds and toast for 2 minutes to become lightly browned and fragrant. Put in a plate and set aside.
2. Put the olive oil, honey, soy sauce, sesame oil, and lime juice, in a small bowl and mix to make the dressing.
3. Put in a large bowl, the kale, cucumber, pak choi, parsley, and red onion and gently mix. Pour the dressing into the mixture and continue mixing.
4. Share the salad in two plates topping them with the shredded chicken. Sprinkle the sesame seeds and serve.

Per serving: Calories: 478 kcal Protein: 19.53 g Fat: 39.8 g Carbohydrates: 12.52 g

Sirtfood Scrambled Eggs

Prep time: 15 minutes

Cook time: 7 minutes

Serves: 2

Ingredients

- 1 tsp extra virgin olive oil

- ¾ oz. red onion, finely chopped
- ½ bird's eye chili, finely chopped
- 3 medium eggs
- 1.7 fl. oz. milk
- 1 tsp ground turmeric
- 3/16 oz. parsley, finely chopped

Method:

1.In a skillet, heat the oil over high heat.

2.Toss in the red onion and chili, frying for 3 minutes.

3.In a large bowl, whisk together the milk, parsley, eggs, and turmeric.

4.Pour into the skillet and lower to medium heat.

5.Cook for 4 minutes, scrambling the mixture as you do with a spoon or spatula.

6.Serve immediately.

Per serving: Calories - 224 Fat - 14.63 g Carbs – 4.79 g Protein – 17.2 g

Chili Artichokes

Prep time: 10 minutes

Cook time: 25 minutes

Serves: 4

Ingredients

- 2 artichokes, trimmed and halved
- 1 teaspoon chili powder
- 2 green chilies, mined
- 2 tablespoons olive oil
- 1 teaspoon garlic powder

•1 teaspoon sweet paprika

•A pinch of salt and black pepper

•Juice of 1 lime

Method:

1.In a roasting pan, combine the artichokes with the chili powder, the chilies and the other ingredients, toss and bake at 380 degrees F for 25 minutes.

2.Divide the artichokes between plates and serve.

Per serving: calories 132, fat 2, fiber 2, carbs 4, protein 6

Not-Tuna Salad

Prep time: 5 Minutes

Cook time: 0 Minutes

Serves: 4

What you need:

- 1 (15.5-ounce) can chickpeas, drained and washed
- 1 (14-ounce) can heart of palm, drained and chopped
- ½ cup chopped yellow or white onion
- ½ cup diced celery
- ¼ cup vegan mayonnaise, plus more if needed
- ½ teaspoon salt
- ¼ teaspoon freshly ground black pepper

Method:

1. Make use of a potato masher or fork to mash the chickpeas until chunky and "shredded roughly." Add the hearts of palm, onion, celery, vegan mayonnaise, salt, and pepper. Combine and add more mayonnaise, if necessary, for a creamy texture.
2. Into each of 4 single-serving containers, place ¾ cup of salad. Seal the lids.

Per serving: Calories: 214 Fat: 6g Protein: 9g Carbohydrates: 35g Fiber: 8g Sugar: 1g Sodium: 765mg

Morning Egg Sandwiches

Prep time: 10 minutes

Cook time: 10 minutes

Serves: 4

What you need:

- 5 oz. whole-grain bread
- 1 tablespoon sunflower seeds butter
- ¼ teaspoon salt
- 1 avocado, pitted
- 4 eggs

Method:

- Slice the bread into 8 slices.
- Preheat a skillet and add the sunflower seeds butter and melt it well.
- Beat the eggs in the skillet and sprinkle them with the salt.
- Chop the avocado into the medium cubes and mash it well.
- Spread the bread slices with the avocado mash.
- When the eggs are cooked, cool them a little and place on top of the bread slices to make the sandwiches.
- Serve the dish immediately.

Per serving: Calories: 275, Fat: 17.7g, Total Carbs: 21.7g, Sugars: 3.2g, Protein: 11.1g

Quinoa Bowl

Prep time: 10 minutes

Cook time: 15 minutes

Serves: 6

What you need:

- 2 cups quinoa
- 1 cup blueberries
- 1 cup coconut milk, unsweetened
- 2 cups of water
- 2 tablespoons almonds
- 1 teaspoon pistachio
- 2 tablespoons honey

Method:

1. Combine the coconut milk and water together in the saucepan and stir the liquid well.
2. Add the quinoa and close the lid.
3. Cook the mixture on medium heat for 5 minutes.
4. Wash the blueberries carefully and add them to the quinoa mixture.
5. Stir it carefully and continue to cook.
6. Combine the pistachio and almonds together and crush the nuts.
7. Sprinkle the quinoa with the crushed nuts and cook the mixture for 3 minutes more.
8. Add honey and stir the mixture carefully until the honey has dissolved.
9. Transfer to serving bowls and enjoy.
10. Enjoy!

Per serving: Calories: 348, Fat: 14.1g, Total Carbs: 48.3g, Sugars: 9.6g, Protein: 9.6g

Sweet Oatmeal

Prep time: 5 minutes

Cook time: 10 minutes

Serves: 3

What you need:

- 1 cup oatmeal
- 5 apricots
- 1 tablespoon honey
- 1 cup coconut milk, unsweetened
- 1 teaspoon cashew butter
- ¼ teaspoon salt
- ½ cup of water

Method:

1. Combine the coconut milk and oatmeal together in the saucepan and stir the mixture.
2. Add the water and stir it again. Sprinkle the mixture with the salt and close the lid.
3. Cook the oatmeal on medium heat for 10 minutes.
4. Meanwhile, chop the apricots into tiny pieces and combine the chopped fruit with the honey.
5. When the oatmeal is cooked, add cashew butter and fruit mixture.
6. Stir carefully and transfer to serving bowls.
7. Serve immediately.

Per serving: Calories: 336, Fat: 21.2g, Total Carbs: 35.1g, Sugars: 14.0g, Protein: 6.2g

Green Beans and Eggs

Prep time: 10 minutes

Cook time: 15 minutes

Serves: 2

What you need:

- ½ cup green beans
- ¼ teaspoon salt
- 5 eggs
- 1/3 cup skim milk
- 1 bell pepper, seeds removed
- 1 teaspoon olive oil

Method:

- Slice the bell pepper and combine it with the green beans.
- Pour the olive oil in a skillet and transfer the vegetable mixture to the skillet.
- Cook on medium heat for 3 minutes, stirring frequently.
- Meanwhile, beat the eggs in a mixing bowl.
- Sprinkle the egg mixture with the salt and add skim milk. Whisk well.
- Pour the egg mixture over the vegetable mixture and cook for 3 minutes on medium heat.
- Stir the mixture carefully so that the eggs and vegetables are well combined.
- Cook for 4 minutes more.
- Stir again and close the lid.
- Cook the scrambled eggs for 5 minutes more.
- Stir the mixture again.
- Serve it.

Per serving: Calories: 231, Fat: 13.4g, Total Carbs: 9.3g, Sugars: 6.2g, Protein: 16.3g

LUNCH

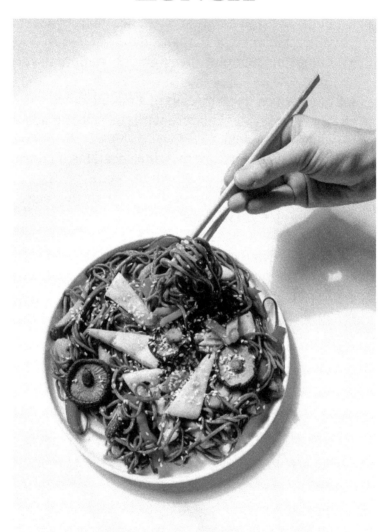

Sticky Chicken Watermelon Noodle Salad

Prep time: 20 minutes

Cook time: 40 minutes

Serves: 2

Ingredients

- 2 pieces of skinny rice noodles
- 1/2 tbsp. sesame oil
- 2 cups watermelon
- Head of bib lettuce
- Half of a lot of scallions
- Half of a lot of fresh cilantro
- 2 skinless, boneless chicken breasts
- 1/2 tbsp. Chinese five-spice
- 1 tbsp. extra virgin olive oil
- Two tbsp. sweet skillet (I utilized a mixture of maple syrup using a dash of tabasco)
- 1 tbsp. sesame seeds
- A couple of cashews - smashed
- Dressing - could be made daily or 2 until
- 1 tbsp. low-salt soy sauce
- 1 teaspoon sesame oil
- 1 tbsp. peanut butter
- Half of a refreshing red chili
- Half of a couple of chives
- Half of a couple of cilantros
- 1 lime - juiced
- 1 small spoonful of garlic

Method:

1. In a bowl, then completely substituting the noodles in boiling drinking water. They are going to be soon spread out in 2 minutes.
2. On a big sheet of parchment paper, throw the chicken with pepper, salt, and the five-spice.

3. Twist over the paper subsequently flattens the chicken using a rolling pin.
4. Place into the large skillet with 1 tbsp. of olive oil, turning 3 or 4 minutes, until well charred and cooked through.
5. Drain the noodles and toss with 1 tbsp. of sesame oil onto a sizable serving dish.
6. Place 50% the noodles into the moderate skillet, frequently stirring until crispy and nice.
7. Remove the watermelon skin, then slice the flesh to inconsistent balls, and then move to plate.
8. Wash the lettuces and cut into small wedges and half of a whole lot of leafy greens and scatter on the dish.
9. Place another 1 / 2 the cilantro pack, the soy sauce, coriander, chives, peanut butter, a dab of water, 1 teaspoon of sesame oil, and the lime juice in a bowl, then mix till smooth.
10. set the chicken back to heat, garnish with all the sweet sauce (or my walnut syrup mixture) and toss with the sesame seeds.
11. Pour the dressing on the salad toss gently with clean fingers until well coated, then add crispy noodles and then smashed cashews.
12. Mix chicken pieces and add them to the salad.

Per serving: Calories: 694 Carbohydrates: 0 Fat: 33g Protein: 0

Fruity Curry Chicken Salad

Prep time: 20 minutes

Cook time: 10 minutes

Serves: 2

Ingredients

- Original recipe yields 8 Serves
- Fixing checklist

- 4 skinless, boneless chicken pliers - cooked and diced
- 1 tsp celery, diced
- 4 green onions, sliced
- 1 golden delicious apple peeled, cored, and diced
- 1/3 cup golden raisins
- 1/3 cup seedless green grapes, halved
- 1/2 cup sliced toasted pecans
- 1/8 Teaspoon ground black pepper
- 1/2 tsp curry powder
- 3/4 cup light mayonnaise

Method:

1. In a big bowl, combine the chicken, onion, celery, apple, celery, celery, pecans, pepper, curry powder, and carrot. Mix altogether. Enjoy!

Per serving: Fat; 44 milligrams Cholesterol: 188 milligrams Sodium. 12.3 g Carbohydrates: 15.1 gram of Protein; full nutrition

Zuppa Toscana

Prep time: 25 minutes

Cook time: 60 minutes

Serves: 2

Ingredients

- 1 lb. ground Italian sausage
- 1 1/4 tsp crushed red pepper flakes
- 4 pieces bacon, cut into ½ inch bits
- 1 big onion, diced
- 1 tbsp. minced garlic
- 5 (13.75 oz.) can chicken broth
- 6 celery, thinly chopped
- 1 cup thick cream
- 1/4 bunch fresh spinach, tough stems removed

Method:

1. Cook that the Italian sausage and red pepper flakes in a pot on medium-high heat until crumbly, browned, with no longer pink, 10 to 15minutes. Drain and put aside.
2. Cook the bacon at the exact Dutch oven over moderate heat until crispy, about 10 minutes. Drain, leaving a couple of tablespoons of drippings together with all the bacon at the bottom of the toaster. Stir in the garlic and onions cook until onions are tender and translucent, about five minutes.
3. Pour the chicken broth to the pot with the onion and bacon mix; contribute to a boil on high temperature. Add the berries and boil until fork-tender, about 20 minutes.
4. Reduce heat to moderate and stir in the cream and the cooked sausage – heat throughout. Mix the lettuce to the soup before serving.

Per serving: Carbohydrates; 32.6 g Fat; 45.8 g Carbs; 19.8 g Protein; 99 Milligrams Cholesterol: 2386

Country Chicken Breasts

Prep time: 10 minutes

Cook time: 45 minutes

Serves: 2

What you need:

•2 medium green apples, diced

•1 small red onion, finely diced

•1 small green bell pepper, chopped

•3 cloves garlic, minced

•2 tablespoons dried currants

•1 tablespoon curry powder

•1 teaspoon turmeric

- 1 teaspoon ground ginger
- ¼ teaspoon chili pepper flakes
- 1 can (14 ½ ounce) diced tomatoes
- 6 skinless, boneless chicken breasts, halved
- ½ cup chicken broth
- 1 cup long-grain white rice
- 1-pound large raw shrimp, shelled and deveined
- Salt and pepper to taste
- Chopped parsley
- 1/3 cup slivered almonds

Method:

1.Rinse chicken, pat dry and set aside.

2.In a large crockpot, combine apples, onion, bell pepper, garlic, currants, curry powder, turmeric, ginger, and chili pepper flakes. Stir in tomatoes.

3.Arrange chicken, overlapping pieces slightly, on top of tomato mixture.

4.Pour in broth and do not mix or stir.

5.Cover and cook at for 6 – 7 hours on low.

6.Preheat oven to 200 degrees F.

7.Carefully transfer chicken to an oven-safe plate, cover lightly, and keep warm in the oven.

8.Stir rice into remaining liquid. Increase cooker heat setting to high; cover and cook, stirring once or twice, until rice is almost tender to bite, 30 to 35 minutes. Stir in shrimp, cover and cook until shrimp are opaque in center, about 10 more minutes.

9.Meanwhile, toast almonds in a small pan over medium heat until golden brown, 5 - 8 minutes, stirring occasionally. Set aside.

10. Mound in a warm serving dish and arrange chicken on top. Sprinkle with parsley and almonds.

Per serving: Calories: 155 Carbs: 13.9g Protein: 17.4g Fat: 3.8g

Apples and Cabbage Mix

Prep time: 5 minutes

Cook time: 0 minutes

Serves: 4

What you need:

• 2 cored and cubed green apples

• 2tbsps. Balsamic vinegar

• ½ tsp. caraway seeds

• 2tbsps. olive oil

• Black pepper

• 1 shredded red cabbage head

Method:

1.In a bowl, combine the cabbage with the apples and the other ingredients, toss and serve.

Per serving: Calories: 165 Fat: 7.4 g Carbs: 26 g Protein: 2.6 g Sugars: 2.6 g Sodium: 19 mg

Rosemary Endives

Prep time: 10 minutes

Cook time: 45 minutes

Serves: 2

What you need:

• 2tbsps. olive oil

• 1 tsp. dried rosemary

- 2 halved endives
- ¼ tsp. black pepper
- ½ tsp. turmeric powder

Method:

1.In a baking pan, combine the endives with the oil and the other ingredients, toss gently, introduce in the oven and bake at 400 0F for 20 minutes.

2.Divide between plates and serve.

Per serving: Calories: 66 Fat: 7.1 g Carbs: 1.2 g Protein: 0.3 g Sugars: 1.3 g Sodium: 113 mg

Kale Sauté

Prep time: 10 minutes

Cook time: 35 minutes

Serves: 2

What you need:

- 1 chopped red onion
- 3tbsps. coconut aminos
- 2tbsps. olive oil
- 1 lb. torn kale
- 1 tbsp. chopped cilantro
- 1 tbsp. lime juice
- 2 minced garlic cloves

Method:

1.Heat up a pan with the olive oil over medium heat, add the onion and the garlic and sauté for 5 minutes.

2.Add the kale and the other ingredients, toss, cook over medium heat for 10 minutes, divide between plates and serve.

Per serving: Calories: 200 Fat: 7.1 g Carbs: 6.4 g Protein: 6 g Sugars: 1.6 g Sodium: 183 mg

Roasted Beets

Prep time: 10 minutes

Cook time: 40 minutes

Serves: 2

What you need:

- 2 minced garlic cloves
- ¼ tsp. black pepper
- 4 peeled and sliced beets
- ¼ c. chopped walnuts
- 2tbsps. olive oil
- ¼ c. chopped parsley

Method:

1.In a baking dish, combine the beets with the oil and the other ingredients, toss to coat, introduce in the oven at 420 0F, and bake for 30 minutes.

2.Divide between plates and serve.

Per serving: Calories: 156 Fat: 11.8 g Carbs: 11.5 g Protein: 3.8 g Sugars: 8 g Sodium: 670 mg

Minty Tomatoes and Corn

Prep time: 10 minutes

Cook time: 65 minutes

Serves: 2

What you need:

- 2 c. corn

- 1 tbsp. rosemary vinegar
- 2tbsps. chopped minutest
- 1 lb. sliced tomatoes
- ¼ tsp. black pepper
- 2tbsps. olive oil

Method:

1.In a salad bowl, combine the tomatoes with the corn and the other ingredients, toss and serve.

2.Enjoy!

Per serving: Calories: 230 Fat: 7.2 g Carbs: 11.6 g Protein: 4 g Sugars: 1 g Sodium: 53 mg

Pesto Green Beans

Prep time: 10 minutes

Cook time: 55 minutes

Serves: 2

What you need:

- 2tbsps. olive oil
- 2 tsps. Sweet paprika
- Juice of 1 lemon
- 2tbsps. basil pesto
- 1 lb. trimmed and halved green beans
- ¼ tsp. black pepper
- 1 sliced red onion

Method:

1.Heat up a pan with the oil over medium-high heat, add the onion, stir and sauté for 5 minutes.

2.Add the beans and the rest of the ingredients, toss, cook over medium heat for 10 minutes, divide between plates and serve.

Per serving: Calories: 280 Fat: 10 g Carbs: 13.9 g Protein: 4.7 g Sugars: 0.8 g Sodium: 138 mg

Scallops and Sweet Potatoes

Prep time: 5 minutes

Cook time: 22 minutes

Serves: 4

What you need:

- 1-pound scallops
- ½ teaspoon rosemary, dried
- ½ teaspoon oregano, dried
- 2 tablespoons avocado oil
- 1 yellow onion, chopped
- 2 sweet potatoes, peeled and cubed
- ½ cup chicken stock
- 1 tablespoon cilantro, chopped

Method:

1.Heat a pan with the oil on medium heat, add the onion and sauté for 2 minutes.

2.Add the sweet potatoes and the stock, toss and cook for 10 minutes more.

3.Add the scallops and the remaining ingredients, toss, cook for another 10 minutes, divide everything into bowls and serve.

Per serving: Calories 211 Fat 2 Fiber 4.1 Carbs 26.9 Protein 20.7

Citrus Salmon

Prep time: 10 minutes

Cook time: 45 minutes

Serves: 2

What you need:

- 1 ½ lb. salmon fillet with skin on
- Salt and pepper to taste
- 1 medium red onion, chopped
- 2 tablespoons parsley, chopped
- 2 teaspoons lemon rind, grated
- 2 teaspoons orange rind, grated
- 2 tablespoons extra virgin olive oil
- 1 lemon, sliced thinly
- 1 orange, sliced thinly
- 1 cup vegetable broth

Method:

1. Line your crockpot with parchment paper and top with the lemon slices.

2. Season salmon with salt and pepper and place it on top of lemon.

3. Cover the fish with the onion, parsley and grated citrus rinds and oil over fish. Top with orange slices, reserving a few for garnish.

4. Pour broth around, but not directly overtop, your salmon.

5. Cover and cook on low for 2 hours.

6. Preheat oven to 400 degrees F.

7. When salmon is opaque and flaky, remove from the crockpot carefully using the parchment paper and transfer to a baking sheet. Place in the oven for 5 – 8 minutes to allow the salmon to brown on top.

8. Serve garnished with orange and lemon slices.

Per serving: Calories 294 Fat 3 Fiber 8 Carbs 49 Protein 21

Sage Carrots

Prep time: 10 minutes

Cook time: 25 minutes

Serves: 2

What you need:

• 2 tsps. Sweet paprika

• 1 tbsp. chopped sage

• 2tbsps. olive oil

• 1 lb. peeled and roughly cubed carrots

• ¼ tsp. black pepper

• 1 chopped red onion

Method:

1.In a baking pan, combine the carrots with the oil and the other ingredients, toss and bake at 380 0F for 30 minutes.

2.Divide between plates and serve.

Per serving: Calories: 200 Fat: 8.7 g Carbs: 7.9 g Protein: 4 g Sugars: 19 g Sodium: 268 mg

Moong Dahl

Prep time: 10 minutes

Cook time: 10 minutes

Serves: 4-6

What you need:

• 300g/10oz split mung beans (moong dahl)

• Preferably soaked for a few hours

• 600ml/1pt of water

• 2 tbsp./30g olive oil, butter or ghee

- •1 red onion, finely chopped
- •1-2 tsp coriander seeds
- •1-2 tsp cumin seeds
- •2-4 tsp fresh ginger, chopped
- •1-2 tsp turmeric
- •¼ tsp of cayenne pepper – more if you want it spicy
- •Salt & black pepper to taste

Method:

1.First drain and rinse the split mung beans. Put them in a pan and cover with the water. Bring to the boil and skim off any foam that arises. Turn down the heat, cover and simmer.

2.Meanwhile, heat the oil in a pan and sauté the onion until onion gets soft.

3.Dry fry the coriander and cumin seeds in a heavy-bottomed pan. Fry until they start to pop. Grind them in a pestle and mortar.

4.Add the ground spices to the onions and also add ginger, turmeric and cayenne pepper. Cook for a few minutes.

5.Once the mung beans are almost done, add the onion and spice mix to them. Season it with salt and pepper and cook for a further 10 minutes.

Per serving: Calories 347 Protein 25.73 Fiber 18.06

Macaroni & Cheese with Broccoli

Prep time: 10 minutes

Cook time: 6 minutes

Serves: 6

What you need:

- 3cups whole-wheat macaroni, uncooked
- 1large fresh broccoli crown, chopped

- ¼cup flour
- 2.5cups milk, divided
- 1½cups shredded extra-sharp cheddar cheese
- 2teaspoons Dijon mustard
- ¼teaspoon garlic powder
- ¾teaspoon paprika
- ¼teaspoon salt
- 2teaspoons extra virgin olive oil
- Crumb topping
- Cooking spray
- 3tablespoons dry breadcrumbs
- ¾teaspoon salt
- ¼teaspoon white pepper

Method:

1. Preheat oven to 400° F. Coat a 2-quart baking dish with cooking spray. Bring a large pot of salted water to a boil.
2. When water boils cook macaroni 4 minutes. Add the raw fresh broccoli. Continue cooking for 2 minutes longer until the pasta is slightly undercooked; the broccoli should be bright green and crisp tender.
3. Meanwhile, prepare cheese sauce. Heat 2 cups milk in a medium saucepan over medium-high heat, stirring often until steaming hot. Whisk together the remaining ½ cup cold milk, flour, Dijon mustard, ¾ teaspoon salt and white pepper in a medium bowl until completely smooth. Whisk the flour mixture into the steaming milk and bring to a simmer whisking often until smooth and thickened.
4. Stir the cheese sauce into the pasta. Transfer the pasta mixture into the prepared baking dish. Stir together breadcrumbs, paprika, ¼ teaspoon salt, and garlic powder in a small bowl. Drizzle in olive oil and stir until completely combined. Sprinkle the crumbs over the pasta and transfer to the oven.

Per serving: Energy (calories):397; Fat:7.1g; Carbohydrates:59.9g; Protein:20.5g

Glazed Tofu with Vegetables and Buckwheat

Prep time: 10 minutes.

Cook time: 20 minutes.

Serves: 1.

What you need:

•150g tofu

•1 tablespoon of mirin

•20g Miso paste

•40g green celery stalk

•35g red onion

•120g courgetti

•1 small Thai chili

•1 garlic clove

•1 small piece of ginger

•50g kale

•2 teaspoons sesame seeds

•35g buckwheat

•1 teaspoon turmeric

•2 teaspoons of extra virgin olive oil

•1 teaspoon soy sauce or tamari

Method:

1. Preheat oven to 400 °.
2. In the meantime, mix mirin and miso. Cut the tofu in half lengthwise and divide into two triangles. Briefly marinate the tofu with the mirin/miso paste while preparing the other ingredients.

3. Cut the celery stalks into thin slices, the zucchini into thick rings and the onion into thin rings. Finely chop garlic, ginger and chili. Coarsely chop the kale and stew or blanch briefly.
4. Place the marinated tofu in a small casserole dish, sprinkle with the sesame seeds and bake in the oven for approx. 15 minutes until the marinade has caramelized slightly.
5. In the meantime, cook the buckwheat according to the package instructions and add turmeric to the water.
6. In the meantime, heat the olive oil in a coated pan and add the celery, onion, courgette, chili, ginger and garlic—cook over high heat for one to two minutes, then two to three minutes at low temperature. Add a little water as required.
7. Serve the glazed tofu with vegetables and buckwheat.

Per serving: Calories: 454 Fat: 24.2g. Carbs: 46.5g. Protein: 17.3g.

Tofu with Cauliflower

Prep time: 10 minutes.

Cook time: 50 minutes.

Serves: 1

What you need:

•60g red pepper, seeded

•1 Thai chili, cut in two halves, seeded

•2 cloves of garlic

•1 teaspoon of olive oil

•1 pinch of cumin

•1 pinch of coriander

- Juice of a 1/4 lemon
- 200g tofu
- 200g cauliflower, roughly chopped
- 40g red onions, finely chopped
- 1 teaspoon finely chopped ginger
- 2 teaspoons turmeric
- 30g dried tomatoes, finely chopped
- 20g parsley, chopped

Method:

1. Preheat oven to 400 °. Slice the peppers and put them in an ovenproof dish with chili and garlic. Pour some olive oil over it, add the dried herbs and put it in the oven until the peppers are soft (about 20 minutes). Let it cool down, put the peppers together with the lemon juice in a blender and work it into a soft mass.
2. Cut the tofu in half and divide the halves into triangles. Place the tofu in a small casserole dish, cover with the paprika mixture and place in the oven for about 20 minutes.
3. Chop the cauliflower until the pieces are smaller than a grain of rice.
4. Then, in a small saucepan, heat the garlic, onions, chili and ginger with olive oil until they become transparent. Add turmeric and cauliflower, mix well and heat again. Remove from heat and add parsley and tomatoes, mix well. Serve with the tofu in the sauce.

Per serving: Calories: 197.3 Fat: 9.4 g. Carbohydrate: 19.3 g Protein: 13.5 g

Filled Pita Pockets

Prep time: 20 minutes.

Cook time: 0 minutes.

Serves: 1

What you need:

•You need whole-grain pita bags.

•For a filling with meat:

•80g roasted turkey breast

•25g rocket salad, finely chopped

•20g cheese, grated

•35g cucumbers, small diced

•30g red onions, finely diced

•15g walnuts, chopped

•Dressing of 1 tablespoon balsamic vinegar and 1 tablespoon extra-virgin olive oil

For a vegan filling:

•3 tablespoons hummus

•35g cucumbers, small diced

•30g red onions, finely diced

•25g rocket salad, finely chopped

•15g walnuts, chopped

•Dressing of 1 tablespoon of extra virgin olive oil and some lemon juice

Method:

In both variations, mix all the ingredients, fill the pita pockets with them and marinate them with the dressing.

Per serving: Calories: 120 Fat: 1g. Carbohydrate: 23g. Protein: 21g

Lima Bean Dip with Celery and Crackers

Prep time: 10 minutes.

Cook time: 0 minutes.

Serves: 2

What you need:

•400g Lima beans or white beans from the tin

•3 tablespoons of olive oil

•Juice and zest of half an untreated lemon

•4 spring onions, cut into fine rings

•1 garlic clove, pressed

•1/4 Thai chili, chopped

Method:

1. Drain the beans. Then mix all ingredients with a potato masher to a mass.
2. Serve with green celery sticks and crackers.

Per serving: Calories: 88 Fat: 0.7g. Carbohydrates: 15.7g. Protein: 5.3g.

Spinach and Eggplant Casserole

Prep time: 15 minutes.

Cook time: 55 minutes.

Serves: 3

What you need:

•Eggplant

•Onion slices

•A spoon of olive oil

•450 g spinach (fresh)

•Tomato

•Egg

•60 ml of almond milk

•1 teaspoon lemon juice

•Almond flour

Method:

1. Preheat the oven to 200 ° C.
2. Brush the eggplant and onions with olive oil and fry them in the pan.
3. Place spinach in a large pot, heat over medium heat, then drain the colander.
4. Put the vegetables in a frying pan: first eggplant, then spinach, then onions and tomatoes. Repeat again
5. Beat eggs with almond milk, lemon juice, salt and pepper, then pour them on the vegetables.
6. Sprinkle almond flour on a plate and bake for about 30 to 40 minutes.

Per serving: Calories: 139.9 Fat: 6.5 g. Carbohydrate: 21.5 g. Protein: 10.3 g.

Ancient Mediterranean Pizza

Prep time: 45 minutes.

Cook time: 35 minutes.

Serves: 3

What you need:

•120 g tapioca flour

•Teaspoon Celtic sea salt

•1 tablespoon Italian spice mix

•45 grams of coconut flour

•120 ml olive oil (fresh) water (hot) 120 ml

•Cover with eggs (slap):

•1 tablespoon tomato paste (can)

•1/2 slices zucchini

•1/2 eggplant

•Tomato slices

•A spoon of olive oil (delicate)

•Balsamic vinegar

Method:

1. Preheat the oven to 190 ° C and cover the pan with parchment paper.
2. Cut the vegetables into thin slices.
3. Put cassava flour and salt, Italian herbs and coconut flour together in a large bowl.
4. Pour olive oil and hot water and mix well.
5. Then add the eggs and stir until the dough is even.
6. If the dough is too thin, add 1 tablespoon of coconut flour at a time until it reaches the desired thickness. Wait a few minutes before adding more coconut flour, as this will take some time to absorb the water. The purpose is to obtain a soft dough.
7. Divide the dough in half, then wrap it in a circle on the baking sheet (or make a large pizza as shown).
8. Bake for 10 minutes.
9. Brush the pizza with tomato sauce, then sprinkle the eggplant, zucchini and tomatoes on the pizza.
10. Pour the pancakes in olive oil and cook for 10 to 15 minutes.
11. Pour balsamic vinegar on pizza before eating.

Per serving: Calories:221.8 Fat:8.0 Carbs: 31g Protein: 12g

Vegetarian Ratatouille

Prep time: 20 minutes.

Cook time: 1 hour.

Serves: 1

What you need:

•200 grams diced tomatoes (canned)

•2 slices onion

•Clove garlic

- •4 teaspoons dried oregano
- •4 c. 1 teaspoon paprika
- •A spoon of olive oil
- •Eggplant
- •Zucchini slices
- •Pepper
- •1 teaspoon dried thyme

Method:

1. Preheat the oven to 180 ° C, then gently lubricate the circle or oval.
2. Finely chop onion and garlic.
3. Mix tomato slices with garlic, onion, oregano and pepper, season with salt and pepper, then put in the bottom of the pot.
4. Use a mandolin, cheese slicer or sharp knife to cut eggplant, zucchini and pepper.
5. Place the vegetables in a bowl (wrapped, starting at the edge and processing inside).
6. Place olive oil on vegetables and sprinkle with thyme, salt and pepper.
7. Cover the pan with parchment paper and bake for 45 to 55 minutes.
8. Please enjoy!

Per serving: Calories: 130 Fat: 1g Carbs: 8g Protein:1g

Spicy Spare Ribs with Roasted Pumpkin

Prep time: 1 day.

Cook time: 1 hour and 15 minutes.

Serves: 5

What you need:

- •400g pork ribs

- A spoon of coconut amino acids
- Honey spoon
- A spoon of olive oil
- 50 g shallots
- Garlic clove
- Green paper
- 1 slice onion
- 1 red pepper
- 1 red pepper

For the roasted pumpkin:

- 1 slice of pumpkin
- 1 tablespoon coconut oil
- 1 teaspoon of chili powder

Method:

1. Pickled pork ribs the day before yesterday.
2. Cut the ribs into four small pieces: mix coconut amino acids, honey and olive oil in a bowl. Chopped green onions, garlic and peppers, then add. Spread the ribs on the plastic container and pour the marinade. Place them in the refrigerator overnight.
3. Cut onions, peppers and peppers into small pieces and place in a slow cooker. Spare ribs (including marinade) and cook for at least 4 hours.
4. Preheat the pumpkin to 200 ° C.
5. Cut the pumpkin on the moon and place it on a baking sheet lined with parchment paper.
6. Place a spoonful of coconut oil on the baking sheet and season with chili, pepper and salt. Roast the pumpkin in the oven for about 20 minutes, and then serve it with the ribs.

Per serving: Calories: 282 Fat: 18g. Carbs:16g. Protein: 12g.

Roast Beef with Grilled Vegetables

Prep time: 20 minutes.

Cook time: 1 hour and 10 minutes.

Serves: 5

What you need:

- 500 g roast beef
- Garlic clove (squeezed)
- One teaspoon fresh rosemary
- 400 g broccoli
- 200g carrots
- 400 g zucchini
- A spoonful of olive oil

Method:

1. Rub roast beef with sweet pepper, salt, garlic and rosemary.
2. Heat the pan over high heat and fry the meat for about 20 minutes, or until brown spots appear on all sides of the flesh.
3. Then wrap it with aluminum foil and let it sit for a while.
4. Before serving, slice the roast beef into thin slices.
5. Preheat the oven to 205 ° C. Put all the vegetables in the pan.
6. Season the vegetables with a little olive oil and then season with curry and paprika. Bake for 30 minutes or until the vegetables are cooked.

Per serving: Calories: 347.6 Fat: 8.0g Carbs: 31g Protein: 32.2

Turkey meatball skewers

Prep time: 5 minutes

Cook time: 75 minutes

Serves: 4

What you need:

•4 sticks of lemongrass

•400g minced turkey

•2 cloves of garlic, finely chopped

•1 egg

•1 red chili, finely chopped

•2 tablespoons lime juice

•2 tablespoons chopped coriander

•1 teaspoon turmeric

•Pepper

Method:

1.Clean lemon grass cut in half lengthwise and wash.

2.Mix the meat with the egg, chili, garlic, coriander, olive oil, lime juice, turmeric and a little pepper. Make little balls out of them.

3.Put the balls on the lemongrass skewer and grill them as you like. Cook them in the oven or fry them in the pan until the balls are ready. A small salad goes with it.

Per serving: Calories 280.0 Fat 35 g Cholesterol 340 mg Fiber 3 g Protein 2.6g

Buckwheat and nut loaf

Prep time: 15 minutes

Cook time: 30 minutes

Serves: 4

What you need:

•225g/8oz buckwheat

•2 tbsp. olive oil

- 225g/8oz mushrooms
- 2-3 carrots, finely diced
- 2-3 tbsp. fresh herbs, finely chopped e.g., oregano, marjoram, thyme and parsley
- 225g/8oz nuts e.g., hazelnuts, almonds, walnuts
- 2 eggs, beaten (or 2 tbsp. tahini for vegan version)
- Salt and pepper

Method:

1. First of all, put the buckwheat in a pan with 350ml/1.5 cups of water and a pinch of salt. Boil it.

2. Cover and simmer with the lid on until all the water has been absorbed – about 10-15 minutes.

3. Meanwhile, sauté the mushrooms and carrots in the olive oil until soft.

4. Blitz the nuts in the food processor until well chopped.

5. Combine the vegetables, cooked buckwheat, herbs and chopped nuts and stir in the eggs. If using tahini instead of eggs combine this with some water to create a thick pouring consistency before stirring it into the buckwheat.

6. Season it with salt and pepper.

7. Transfer to a lined or oiled loaf tin and bake in the oven on gas mark 5/190C for 30 minutes until set and just browning on top.

Per serving: Calories 163 Carbs 23g Protein 6g Fiber 4g

Almond Butter and Alfalfa Wraps

Prep time: 10 minutes

Cook time: 10 minutes

Serves: 3

What you need:

- 4 tbsp. of almond nut butter

- Juice of 1 lemon
- 2-3 carrots – grated
- 3 radishes, finely sliced
- 1 cup of alfalfa sprouts
- Salt and pepper
- Lettuce leaves or nori sheets

Method:

1.First, mix the almond butter with most of the lemon juice and enough water to make a creamy consistency. Now combine the grated carrot, alfalfa sprouts in a bowl. Sprinkle them with the rest of the lemon juice and season with salt and pepper.

2.Spread the lettuce leaves or nori sheets with almond butter and top with the carrot and sprout mixture. Roll up and eat immediately!

Per serving: Calories: 266

Roast Chicken and Broccoli

Prep time: 15 minutes.

Cook time: 35 minutes.

Serves: 3

What you need:

- A spoon of coconut oil
- 400 g bacon chicken 150 g
- Broccoli 250g

Method:

1. Cut the chicken into squares.
2. Melt coconut oil in a pan over medium heat, brown the chicken and bacon, then cook.
3. Add chili powder, salt and pepper to taste.
4. Add broccoli and brown it.

5. Heap is fun!

Per serving: Calories: 241.3 Fat: 10.9 g. Carbohydrate: 8.5 g Protein: 29.6 g.

Stuffed Eggplant

Prep time: 10 minutes.

Cook time: 1 hour and 20 minutes.

Serves: 3

What you need:

•Eggplant

•A spoon of coconut oil

•Onion slices

•250 grams minced meat

•Clove garlic

•Tomato slices

•1 tablespoon tomato paste

•1 caper manually

•Fresh basil

Method:

1. Finely chop onion and garlic. Cut the tomatoes into small pieces and chop the basil leaves.
2. Bring the kettle to a boil, add the eggplant and cook for about 5 minutes.
3. Drain the water to allow it to cool a little, then use a spoon to remove the flesh (leaving a margin of about 1 cm on the skin). Destroy the pulp and set it aside.
4. Place the eggplant in the pan.
5. Preheat the oven to 175 ° C.
6. Heat 3 tablespoons of coconut oil in a pan over low heat, then coat the onions with a layer of onions.

7. Add ground beef and garlic, then fry until the beef melts.
8. Add chopped eggplant, tomato slices, capers, basil and tomato sauce, and fry in a covered pan for 10 minutes.
9. Season with salt and pepper.
10. Add the beef mixture to the eggplant and fry in the oven for about 20 minutes.

Per serving: Calories: 310.7 Fat: 9.0g Carbs 31g Protein: 26.8g

Parmesan Chicken and Kale Sauté

Prep time: 5 minutes.

Cook time: 10 minutes.

Serves: 6.

What you need:

•Chicken breasts, boneless and skinless – 1.5 pounds

•Extra virgin olive oil – 2 tablespoons

•Sea salt – 1 teaspoon

•Onion, diced – 1

•Red pepper flakes – .25 teaspoon

•Lemon juice – 1 tablespoon

•Black pepper, ground – .25 teaspoon

•Garlic, minced – 3 cloves

•Chicken broth – .5 cup

•Parmesan cheese, grated – .5 cup

•Kale, chopped – 12 ounces

Method:

1. Slice the chicken breasts into long strips, each half an inch thick.

2. Add the extra virgin olive oil to a large skillet and set the stove to medium heat. Allow the olive oil to heat until it shimmers, but don't let it smoke. Add the chicken, sea salt, and black pepper, sautéing it until the chicken is fully cooked through, about five to seven minutes. The chicken breasts are ready when they reach an internal temperature of Fahrenheit one-hundred and sixty-five degrees.
3. Transfer the cooked chicken breast to a plate and cover it with aluminum or a lid to keep it warm.
4. Add the minced garlic, diced onion, and red pepper flakes to the now-empty skillet, sautéing for about two minutes until the onions soften.
5. Add the kale and broth to the skillet and then cover with a lid. Stir occasionally, allowing the kale to cook until tender, about five minutes.
6. Add the cooked chicken breast back into the skillet along with the lemon juice and Parmesan cheese. Stir everything to combine and then remove the skillet from the heat before serving.

Per serving: kcal: 261. Calories: 261. Fat: 24g. Carbs: 30g. Protein: 28g.

The Bell Pepper Fiesta

Prep time: 10 minutes

Cook time: 0 minutes

Serves: 4

What you need:

•2 tablespoons dill, chopped

•1 yellow onion, chopped

•1 pound multi colored peppers, cut, halved, seeded and cut into thin strips

•3 tablespoons organic olive oil

•2 ½ tablespoons white wine vinegar

•Black pepper to taste

Method:

1.Take a bowl and mix in sweet pepper, onion, dill, pepper, oil, vinegar and toss well.

2.Divide between bowls and serve.

3.Enjoy!

Per serving: Calories: 120 Fat: 3g Carbohydrates: 1g Protein: 6g

Spiced Up Pumpkin Seeds Bowls

Prep time: 10 minutes

Cook time: 20 minutes

Serves: 4

What you need:

•½ tablespoon chili powder

•½ teaspoon cayenne

•2 cups pumpkin seeds

•2 teaspoons lime juice

Method:

1.Spread pumpkin seeds over lined baking sheet; add lime juice, cayenne and chili powder.

2.Toss well.

3.Pre-heat your oven to 275 degrees F.

4.Roast in your oven for 20 minutes and transfer to small bowls.

5.Serve and enjoy!

Per serving: Calories: 170 Fat: 3g Carbohydrates: 10g Protein: 6g

Chicken & Bean Casserole

Prep time: 5 Minutes

Cook time: 40 Minutes

Serves: 2

What you need:

•400g 14oz chopped tomatoes

•400g 14 oz. tinned cannellini beans or haricot beans

•8 chicken thighs, skin removed

•2 carrots, peeled and finely chopped

•2 red onions, chopped

•4 sticks of celery

•4 large mushrooms

•2 red peppers bell peppers, deseeded and chopped

•1 clove of garlic

•2 tablespoons soy sauce

•1 tablespoon olive oil

•1.75 liters 3 pints chicken stock broth

•509 calories per serving

Method:

1.Heat the olive oil. Add the garlic and onions and cook for 5 minutes.

2.Add in the chicken, carrots, cannellini beans, celery, red peppers bell peppers and mushrooms.

3.Pour in the stock broth soy sauce and tomatoes.

4.Bring it to the boil. Serve.

Per serving: Calories: 330 Cal Fat: 25 g Carbs: 32 g Protein: 16 g Fiber: 20 g

Mussels in Red Wine Sauce

Prep time: 5 Minutes

Cook time: 50 Minutes

Serves: 2

What you need:

•800g 2lb mussels

•2 x 400g 14 oz. tins of chopped tomatoes

•25g 1oz butter

•1 tablespoon fresh chives, chopped

•1 tablespoon fresh parsley, chopped

•1 bird's-eye chili, finely chopped

•4 cloves of garlic, crushed

•400 ml 14fl. oz. red wine

•Juice of 1 lemon

Method:

1.Heat the butter in a large saucepan and add in the red wine.

2.Reduce the heat and add the parsley, chives, chili and garlic whilst stirring.

3.Add in the tomatoes, lemon juice and mussels.

4.Cover the saucepan and cook for 2-3 minutes.

5.Serve.

Per serving: Calories: 364 Cal Fat: 5 g Carbs: 26 g Protein: 16 g Fiber: 15 g

DINNER

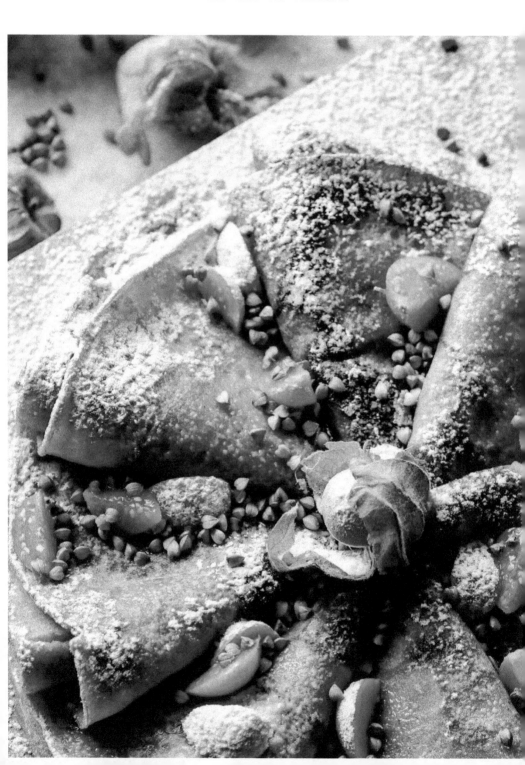

Spiced Cauliflower Couscous with Chicken

Prep time: 15 minutes

Cook time: 20 minutes

Serves: 2

What you need:

- 2 cups roughly chopped cauliflower florets
- A handful fresh flat-leaf parsley
- 2 cloves garlic, finely chopped
- ½ cup finely chopped red onions
- 2 teaspoons finely chopped ginger
- 1/3 cup sun-dried tomatoes
- 2 tablespoons capers
- 2 chicken breasts
- 4 teaspoons turmeric powder
- ½ cup finely diced carrots
- 2 bird's eye chilies, finely chopped
- 4 tablespoons extra-virgin olive oil
- Juice of a lemon

Method:

1. You can chop the cauliflower in a food processor.

2. Place a pan over medium – high flame. Add 2 tablespoons oil. When the oil is heated, add ginger, garlic and chili and cook for a few seconds until fragrant.

3. Stir in turmeric and cook for 5 – 8 seconds. Stir in the carrots and cauliflower and cook for about 2 minutes. Turn off the heat.

4. Transfer into a bowl. Add tomatoes and parsley and stir. Keep warm.

5.Add remaining oil into the pan and let it heat. Place chicken in the pan and cook for about 6 minutes. Turn the chicken over and cook for 5 – 6 minutes or until well-cooked inside.

6.Stir in capers, lemon juice and a sprinkle of water.

7.Add cauliflower and carrot mixture and toss well.

8.Serve.

Per serving: Calories: 250 Fat: 4.5g Protein: 68g Total Carbohydrates: 13g Dietary Fiber: 5g Sodium: 532mg

Chicken Noodles

Prep time: 10 minutes

Cook time: 30 minutes

Serves: 8 – 10

What you need:

•16 ounces buckwheat noodles

•2 yellow bell peppers, chopped into ½ inch squares

•6 cloves garlic, chopped

•2 tablespoons olive oil

•6 cups tomato sauce

•2 tablespoons fresh basil, chopped or 2 teaspoons dry basil

•2 tablespoons fresh parsley, chopped or 2 teaspoons dried parsley

•Pepper to taste

•2 pounds skinless, boneless chicken breast, cut into strips

•1 large red onion, chopped into ½ inch squares, separate the layers

•Salt to taste

Method:

1.Follow the directions on the package and cook the buckwheat noodles.

2.Place a large skillet over medium flame. Add oil and wait for the oil to heat. Add chicken strips and spread it all over the pan and cook undisturbed, until the underside is cooked. Flip sides and cook the other side, undisturbed.

3.Add the vegetables and mix well. Cook until the vegetables are tender. Add tomato sauce and cook for 7-8 minutes.

4.Add noodles and toss well.

5.Serve hot.

Per serving: Calories 372.3 Total Fat 12.4 g Protein 42.6 g Carbs 26.1 g

Aromatic Chicken Breast with Kale, Red Onion and Salsa

Prep time: 10 minutes

Cook time: 20 minutes

Serves: 2

What you need:

•ounces skinless, boneless chicken breasts

•2 teaspoons lemon juice

•ounces kale leaves, chopped

•2 teaspoons minced fresh ginger

•4 teaspoons turmeric powder

•2 tablespoons extra-virgin olive oil

•medium red onion, sliced

•ounces buckwheat groats

For salsa:

•tomatoes, finely chopped

- chili, sliced
- tablespoon capers
- teaspoons lemon juice
- ¼ cup minced parsley
- Salt to taste

Method:

1. To make salsa: Combine tomatoes, chili, capers, lemon juice, parsley and salt into a bowl and toss well. Cover and set aside for a while for the flavors to set in.
2. Sprinkle 2 teaspoons turmeric powder over the chicken. Drizzle lemon juice and a little over it.
3. Place an ovenproof pan over medium flame. Add a little oil. When the oil is heated, add chicken and cook until light golden brown all over.
4. Shift the pan into an oven preheated to 450° F and bake for about 20 minutes or well-cooked inside.
5. Remove the pan from the oven and tent loosely with foil.
6. Meanwhile, steam kale for 5 minutes in the steaming equipment you have.
7. Also cook the buckwheat noodles following the directions on the package, adding remaining turmeric while cooking.
8. Place a skillet over medium flame. Add some oil. When the oil is heated, add onion and ginger and cook until slightly tender.
9. Stir in kale and cook for a minute.
10. Serve chicken with vegetables with salsa on the side.

Per serving: Total Fat 1. 5g Saturated Fat 0g Trans Fat 0g Total Carbs 29.5g Fiber 3g Protein 18.

Chicken Butternut Squash Pasta

Prep time: 10 minutes

Cook time: 30 – 40 minutes

Serves: 2

What you need:

- ½ pound ground chicken
- tablespoon balsamic vinegar
- ½ tablespoon olive oil, divided
- ½ cups whole wheat pasta
- Pepper to taste
- fresh basil leaves, thinly sliced
- tablespoons chopped walnuts
- Salt to taste
- ½ cups cubed butternut squash, cut into ½" cubes
- ounces goat's cheese, crumbled
- ½ teaspoon garlic, minced
- 1/8 teaspoon ground nutmeg

Method:

1 Place butternut squash on a baking sheet. Drizzle 1 tablespoon oil and sprinkle salt and pepper over the squash. Toss well.

2 Bake squash in an oven preheated to 400° F, for about 30 minutes or until tender.

3 Cook the pasta following the directions on the package.

4 Place a skillet over medium heat. Add ½ tablespoon oil and wait for it to heat. Add garlic and cook until light brown, stirring often.

5 Add chicken and cook until the chicken is not pink anymore.

6 Stir in walnuts, nutmeg and vinegar.

7 Cook on low heat for 1 – 2 minutes.

8 Serve chicken over pasta.

9 Scatter butternut squash and goat's cheese. Sprinkle basil on top.

10 Serve.

Per serving: Sodium: 198 mg Cholesterol: 0.0 mg Total Carbs: 39.0 g Fiber: 15.0 g Protein: 12.0 g Calories: 247.0

Chicken Marsala

Prep time: 10 minutes

Cook time: 30 – 40 minutes

Serves: 8

What you need:

•8 boneless, skinless chicken breasts (6 ounces each)

•20 ounces cremini mushrooms, sliced

•2 cloves garlic, peeled, sliced

•1 cup marsala wine

•6 tablespoons flour

•2 large shallots, chopped

•Salt to taste

•1 cup chicken broth

•Freshly ground pepper to taste

•4 – 5 tablespoons olive oil

•2 tablespoons chopped parsley

•Sautéed spinach to serve

Method:

1.Place the chicken breasts between 2 sheets of plastic wrap and pound with a meat mallet until ½ inch in thickness.

2.Sprinkle salt and pepper over the chicken. Sprinkle flour over the chicken.

3.Place a large skillet over medium flame. Add about a tablespoon of oil and swirl the pan to spread the oil.

4.Place as many chicken pieces as possible in the pan. Sear the chicken on both the sides until golden brown. Remove the chicken from the pan placed on a plate using a slotted spoon.

5.Cook the remaining chicken in the same way, adding more oil if required.

6.Add 2 tablespoons oil into the skillet. When the oil is heated, add mushrooms and cook until brown.

7.Stir in garlic and shallots. Add salt and pepper to taste and stir-fry for 1 – 2 minutes.

8.Add wine, broth and chicken along with the released juice and cook until the liquid in the pan is half its original quantity.

9.Garnish with parsley and serve along with sautéed spinach or any other sautéed greens of your choice.

Per serving: Calories: 90 Sodium: 20mg Fat: 3g Cholesterol: 2mg Carbohydrates: 11g Protein: 3g

Chicken Skewers with Satay Sauce

Prep time: 60 minutes

Cook time: 30 minutes

Serves: 2

What you need:

For chicken:

•10.5 ounces chicken breasts, chopped into chunks

•1 teaspoon extra-virgin olive oil

•A handful kale leaves, discard stems and ribs, sliced

•2 teaspoons turmeric powder

For satay sauce:

•2 teaspoons extra-virgin olive oil

- •1 medium red onion, diced
- •2 stalks celery, sliced
- •2 teaspoons curry powder
- •½ cup chicken stock
- •2 tablespoons walnut butter or peanut butter
- •1 ¼ cups coconut milk
- •2 teaspoons turmeric powder
- •2 cloves garlic, peeled, chopped
- •Salt to taste
- •A handful fresh cilantro, chopped

To serve:

- •8 walnut halves, chopped, to garnish
- •3.5 ounces buckwheat

Method:

1. Combine olive oil and turmeric powder in a bowl. Add chicken and stir until chicken is well coated with the mixture. Cover and set aside for about an hour.
2. Meanwhile, follow the directions on the package and cook the buckwheat. Add kale and celery during the last 5 minutes of cooking.
3. Set up your grill and preheat it to high.
4. To make satay sauce: Place a pan over medium flame. Add oil and let it heat. Add onion and garlic and cook for a few minutes until onions turn pink.
5. Stir in turmeric and curry powder and cook for a few more seconds.
6. Pour stock and coconut milk and mix well. When the mixture comes to a boil, stir in the walnut butter. Mix until well combined.
7. Lower the heat and simmer until sauce is thick. Turn off the heat. Add cilantro and stir.

8. While the sauce is thickening, insert the chicken on 2 skewers.
9. Grill the chicken for 10 minutes. Turn the skewers every 3 – 4 minutes.
10. Place the skewers on individual serving plates.
11. Drizzle sauce over the skewers. Scatter walnuts on top and serve.

Per serving: Calories: 55 Fat: 2 g Sodium: 83 mg Carbohydrates: 0 g Protein: 2 g

Turkey Steak with Spicy Cauliflower Couscous

Prep time: 10 minutes

Cook time: 15 – 18 minutes

Serves: 2 – 3

What you need:

- 2 – 3 turkey steaks
- ½ red onion, chopped
- tablespoon ground turmeric
- Juice of ½ lemon
- Olive oil, as required
- ½ cauliflower, chopped to couscous like texture
- Bird's eye chili, chopped
- Salt to taste
- ½ cup chopped parsley
- clove garlic, peeled, minced
- Pepper to taste

Method:

1. Sprinkle salt, pepper and lemon juice over the steaks.
2. Place a pan over medium flame. Add a little oil and let it heat. Add onion, garlic and chili and cook until slightly pink.

85

3. Stir in the turmeric and cauliflower. Heat thoroughly. Turn off the heat. Stir in parsley.
4. Cook the steaks on a preheated grill or in a grill pan.
5. Divide cauliflower couscous into 2 – 3 plates. Top each with a steak and serve.

Per serving: Calories: 56 Fat: 2 g Sodium: 83 mg Carbohydrates: 0 g Fiber: 0 g Protein: 2 g

Turkey Apple Burgers

Prep time: 15 minutes

Cook time: 8 – 10 minutes

Serves: 2

What you need:

•1 green apple, cored, peeled, halved

•A handful fresh thyme or sage, minced

•Pepper to taste

•½ teaspoon onion powder

•¼ teaspoon garlic powder

•Salt to taste

•1 teaspoon olive oil

•½ pound 93% lean ground turkey

•Whole-wheat burger buns or lettuce cups to serve

Method:

1. Grate one half of the apple and cut the other half into thin slices.
2. Combine grated apple, spices, salt, sage and turkey in a bowl and mix well.
3. Make 2 equal portions of the mixture. Shape into patties.
4. Place a skillet over medium flame. Brush oil on both the sides of the patties and place in the pan.

5. Cook until the underside is brown. Turn the burgers over and cook the other side until brown.
6. Serve burgers over buns or lettuce cups. Place sliced apples on top of the burgers and serve.

Per serving: Calories: 10 218 215 Total Fat: 15 613 Saturated Fat: 3753 Sodium: 1342 Total Carbohydrate: Protein: 121

Turkey Sandwiches with Apple and Walnut Mayo

Prep time: 15 minutes

Cook time: 4 minutes

Serves: 2

What you need:

For walnut mayonnaise:

•2 tablespoons finely chopped walnuts

•3 – 4 tablespoons mayonnaise

•½ tablespoon Dijon mustard

•½ tablespoon chopped, fresh parsley

For sandwich:

•4 slices whole-wheat bread

•½ green apple, peeled, cored, cut into thin slices

•Cooked, sliced turkey, as required

•A handful rockets

Method:

1. To make walnut mayonnaise: Combine walnuts, mayonnaise, mustard and parsley in a bowl.
2. Smear walnut mayonnaise on one side of the bread slices.
3. Place arugula on 2 bread slices, on the mayo side. Place turkey slices over it followed by apple slices.

4. Complete the sandwich by covering with remaining bread slices, with mayo side facing down.
5. Cut into desired shape and serve.

Per serving: Calories: 205 Protein: 5.2g Carbs: 30.7g Fat: 12.1g Sodium: 66. 5mg

Sautéed Turkey with Tomatoes and Cilantro

Prep time: 10 minutes

Cook time: 15 minutes

Serves: 2 – 3

What you need:

• ½ pound lean ground turkey

• ½ cup chopped yellow or red onion

• Pepper to taste

• 1 teaspoon olive oil

• 1 jalapeño or to taste, chopped

• ½ tablespoon minced garlic

• ¼ cup chopped tomatoes

• ¼ teaspoon ground cumin

• 2 teaspoons red pepper flakes

• ½ cup chopped fresh cilantro

• Salt to taste

• A handful parsley leaves

Method:

1. Place a skillet over medium flame. Add oil and wait for it to heat. Add garlic and sauté for about a minute until light brown.
2. Stir in onions, tomatoes, jalapeño, parsley and red pepper flakes and cook for 4-5 minutes.

3. Stir in the turkey and cook until brown, breaking the turkey as it cooks.
4. Add cilantro, salt and pepper and stir.
5. Serve hot.

Per serving: Calories: 416 cal. – kcal: 1750 - Fat: 19 g - Protein: 45 g - Carbs: 28 g - Sodium: 171.5 mg

Chargrilled Beef with Red Wine Jus, Onion Rings, Garlic Kale and Herb Roasted Potatoes

Prep time: 10 minutes

Cook time: 1 hour and 30 minutes

Serves: 2

What you need:

•7 ounces potatoes, peeled, cut into 1-inch cubes

•A handful fresh parsley, chopped

•½ ounce kale leaves, chopped, discard hard stems and ribs

•2 beef fillet steaks (4 – 5 ounces each) or 1-inch thick sirloin steak

•¼ cup beef stock

•Salt to taste

•½ teaspoons cornstarch mixed with 2 tablespoons water

•½ tablespoons extra-virgin olive oil

•medium red onion, cut into thin rings

•cloves garlic, finely chopped

•Pepper to taste

•tablespoons red wine

•2 teaspoons tomato puree

Method:

1.Boil water in a saucepan over high flame. Add potatoes and let it come to a rolling boil. Cook for 4 minutes. Drain in a colander.

2.Transfer the potatoes into a baking dish. Drizzle a tablespoon of oil over the potatoes and toss well. Spread it evenly.

3.Bake in an oven preheated to 440° F, for about 30 – 40 minutes. Stir the potatoes at intervals of 10 minutes.

4.Transfer into a bowl. Add parsley and toss well.

5.Place a skillet over medium flame. Add ½ tablespoon oil. When the oil is heated, add onion and cook until golden brown. Transfer into a bowl.

6.Steam kale in the steaming equipment you have.

7.Add ½ tablespoon oil into the skillet. Add garlic and cook for a few seconds until fragrant. Stir in the kale and cook for a couple of minutes, until it turns slightly limp. Turn off the heat. Cover and set aside.

8.Place an ovenproof pan over high-high flame. Add remaining oil and wait for the oil to heat. Once the oil is heated, add steaks and coat it with oil, on both the sides. Cook for 3 to 4 minutes on each side. Turn off the heat.

9.Shift the saucepan into an oven preheated to 440° F, and roast until the meat is cooked to the desired doneness.

10.Take out the pan from the oven. Set the meat aside on a plate.

11.Pour red wine into the same pan. Deglaze the pan. Place the pan over high flame. Cook until the wine is half its original quantity.

12.Stir in stock, tomato puree, and let it come to a boil.

13.Stir in the corn flour mixture. Keep stirring until thick. Pour any cooked juices of the steak into the pan.

14.Serve steak with potatoes, kale, wine sauce and onions.

Per serving: Calories: 570 % Total Fat 42.0g Cholesterol 110.0mg Sodium 980.0mg Carbohydrates 11.0g

Orecchiette with Sausage and Chicory

Prep time: 10 minutes

Cook time: 20 – 25 minutes

Serves: 3

What you need:

- ½ pound Orecchiette
- ½ pound sweet Italian sausage, discard casings
- ¼ teaspoon crushed red pepper
- Salt to taste
- 2 tablespoons grated pecorino + extra to garnish
- 2 tablespoons extra-virgin olive oil
- 1 clove garlic, peeled, thinly sliced
- ½ pound chicory or escarole, chopped
- ½ cup chicken stock
- A handful fresh mint leaves, chopped

Method:

1. Cook pasta following the directions on the package, adding salt while cooking.

2. Place a large skillet over medium flame. Add a tablespoon of oil and let it heat.

3. Once oil is heated, add sausage and cook until brown. Break it while it cooks.

4. Remove sausage with a slotted spoon and place on a plate.

5. Add a tablespoon of oil. When the oil is heated, add garlic and red pepper and stir for a few seconds until you get a nice aroma.

6. Stir in chicory and salt and cook covered, until they turn limp. It should take a couple of minutes.

7. Uncover and continue cooking until tender.

8.Add pasta, sausage, cheese and stock and cook until the sauce is slightly thick. Add mint and stir.

9.Serve hot.

Per serving: 700 Calories 46 g Protein 25 g Carbohydrate 21 g Fat 14 g Saturated Fat 12 mg Cholesterol 93 mg Sodium

Chili Con Carne

Prep time: 15 minutes

Cook time: 1 hour and 30 minutes

Serves: 8

What you need:

•2 red onions, finely chopped

•4 bird's eye chili, finely chopped

•2 red bell peppers, cut into 1-inch squares

•6 cloves garlic, finely chopped

•2 tablespoons extra-virgin olive oil

•1.8 pounds lean, minced beef

•4 cans (14.1 ounces each) chopped tomatoes

•¼ cups red wine

•tablespoons tomato puree

•tablespoons turmeric powder

•2 tablespoons cocoa powder

•2 tablespoons ground cumin

•Pepper to taste

•ounces canned or cooked kidney beans

•A handful fresh parsley, chopped

•A handful fresh cilantro, chopped

•cups beef stock

•ounces buckwheat groats

•Salt to taste

Method:

1.Place a Dutch oven over medium flame. Add oil and wait for it to heat. Add onion, chilies and garlic and cook until slightly soft.

2.Stir in turmeric and cumin.

3.After about 10 – 15 seconds, stir in the beef and raise the heat to high. Cook until brown.

4.Stir in wine and deglaze the pot. Cook until wine reduces to half its original quantity.

5.Stir in bell pepper, cocoa, tomato puree, kidney beans and tomatoes and mix well.

6.Cook covered, on low heat for about an hour. Add some water if at any time you find that the mixture is very thick.

7.While the chili is simmering, follow the directions on the package and cook the buckwheat.

8.Serve chili over buckwheat.

Per serving: 142 Kcal 3.7 Grams Healthy Fat 7.5 Grams Protein 12.5 Grams Total Carb 13.7 Grams Fiber 8.3 Grams Sugars 807 MG Sodium

Lamb and Black Bean Chili

Prep time: 10 minutes

Cook time: 1 hour and 30 minutes

Serves: 4

What you need:

•¾ pound lean ground lamb

•1 clove garlic, minced

•½ cup dry red wine

•1 teaspoon ground cumin

- Salt to taste
- Hot sauce to taste (optional)
- ½ cup chopped red onion
- 1 can (14.1 ounces) whole tomatoes, with its liquid, chopped
- ½ tablespoon chili powder
- 1 teaspoon dried oregano
- 1 ½ cans (15 ounces each) black beans, drained
- ½ teaspoon sugar
- Fresh cilantro sprigs (optional)

Method:

1. Place a Dutch oven over medium flame. Add lamb, onion and garlic and sauté until brown. Break it while you stir.

2. Use a slotted spoon to remove the mixture and place it on a board lined with paper towels. Discard the remaining fat in the pan. Wipe the pot clean.

3. Place the pot over medium flame. Add tomatoes, spices, oregano and salt and stir. Heat thoroughly.

4. Lower the heat and cook covered, for an hour. Add beans and hot sauce and stir.

5. Cover and simmer for about 30 minutes.

6. Sprinkle cilantro on top and serve.

Per serving: Calories 270 Fat 13 g Cholesterol 15 mg Sodium 679 mg Potassium 696 mg Carbohydrates 15 g Fiber 6 g Sugar 4 g Protein 19 g

Tomato, Bacon and Arugula Quiche with Sweet Potato Crust

Prep time: 15 minutes

Cook time: 50 minutes

Serves: 8

What you need:

•4 cups shredded sweet potato or yam

•Salt to taste

•1 red onion, chopped

•2 large handfuls baby arugula

•12 eggs

•2 tablespoons olive oil

•8 slices bacon, chopped

•16 cherry tomatoes, quartered

•6 cloves garlic, minced

•Pepper to taste

•1 tablespoon butter or ghee

Method:

1.To make sweet potato crusts: You can grate the sweet potatoes on a box grater or in the food processor.

2.Squeeze excess moisture from the sweet potatoes.

3.Grease 2 pie pans (9 inches each) with some of the olive oil.

4.Add butter, pepper and salt into the bowl of sweet potatoes and mix well. Press the mixture onto the bottom and a little on the sides of the pie pan.

5.Bake the crusts in an oven preheated to 450° F, for around 20 minutes or until golden brown at the edges.

6.Remove the pie crusts from the oven.

7.Meanwhile, place a skillet over medium heat. Add bacon and cook until crisp. Remove the bacon with a slotted spoon and place on a plate lined with paper towels. Discard the fat.

8.Add remaining oil into the skillet. Once oil is heated, add onions and sauté until it turns soft.

9.Stir in tomatoes and arugula and cook until the tomatoes are slightly soft.

10.Add garlic and cook for about half a minute. Turn off the heat. Cool for a while.

11.Meanwhile, crack the eggs into a bowl. Add salt and pepper and whisk well.

12.Add the slightly cooled vegetables and bacon and stir.

13.Divide the egg mixture equally and pour over the baked sweet potato crust.

14.Place the crusts into the oven and bake until the eggs are set.

15.Let it rest for 10 minutes.

16.Cut each into 4 wedges and serve.

Per serving: Calories, 515 fat, 30g total carbohydrate, 6g fiber, 657mg sodium, 99g protein.

Beef Burritos

Prep time: 10 minutes

Cook time: 20 minutes

Serves: 6

What you need:

•¼ cup white onion, chopped

•¼ cup green bell pepper, chopped

•1-pound ground beef

•¼ cup tomato puree, low-sodium

•¼ teaspoon ground black pepper

•¼ teaspoon ground cumin

•6 flour tortillas, burrito size

Method:

1.Take a skillet pan, place it over medium heat and when hot, add beef and cook for 5 to 8 minutes until browned.

2.Drain the excess fat, then transfer beef to a plate lined with paper towels and serve.

3.Return pan over medium heat, grease it with oil and when hot, add pepper and onion and cook for 5 minutes, or until softened.

4.Switch to low heat, return beef to the pan, season with black pepper and cumin, pour in tomato puree, stir until mixed and cook for 5 minutes until done.

5.Distribute beef mixture evenly on top of the tortilla, roll them in burrito style by folding both ends and then serve.

Per serving: Calories: 265 kcal Total Fat: 9 g Saturated Fat: 0 g Cholesterol: 37 mg Sodium: 341 mg Total Carbs: 31 g Fiber: 1.6 g Protein: 15 g

Broccoli and Beef Stir-Fry

Prep time: 5 minutes

Cook time: 18 minutes

Serves: 4

What you need:

•12 ounces frozen broccoli, thawed

•8 ounces sirloin beef, cut into thin strips

•1 medium Roma tomato, chopped

•1 teaspoon minced garlic

•1 tablespoon cornstarch

•2 tablespoons soy sauce, reduced-sodium

•¼ cup chicken broth, low-sodium

•2 tablespoons peanut oil

•2 cups cooked brown rice

Method:

1.Take a frying pan, place it over medium heat, add oil and when hot, add garlic and cook for 1 minute until fragrant.

2.Add vegetable blend, cook for 5 minutes, then transfer vegetable blend to a plate and set aside until needed.

3.Add beef strips into the pan, and then cook for 7 minutes until cooked to the desired level.

4.Prepare the sauce by putting cornstarch in a bowl, and then whisking in soy sauce and broth until well combined.

5.Returned vegetables to the pan, add tomatoes, drizzle with sauce, stir well until coated, and cook for 2 minutes until the sauce has thickened.

6.Serve with brown rice.

Per serving: Calories: 373 kcal Total Fat: 17 g Saturated Fat: 0 g Cholesterol: 42 mg Sodium: 351 mg Total Carbs: 37 g Fiber: 5.1 g Sugar: 0 g Protein: 18 g

Meatballs with Eggplant

Prep time: 15 minutes

Cook time: 60 minutes

Serves: 6

What you need:

•1-pound ground beef

•½ cup green bell pepper, chopped

•2 medium eggplants, peeled and diced

•½ teaspoon minced garlic

•1 cup stewed tomatoes

•½ cup white onion, diced

•1/3 cup canola oil

•1 teaspoon lemon and pepper seasoning, salt-free

•1 teaspoon turmeric

- 1 teaspoon Mrs. Dash seasoning blend
- 2 cups of water

Method:

1.Take a large skillet pan, place it over medium heat, add oil in it and when hot, add garlic and green bell pepper and cook for 4 minutes until sauté.

2.Transfer green pepper mixture to a plate, set aside until needed then eggplant pieces into the pan and cook for 4 minutes per side until browned, and when done, transfer eggplant to a plate and set aside until needed.

3.Take a medium bowl, place beef in it, add onion, season with all the spices, stir until well combined, and then shape the mixture into 30 small meatballs.

4.Place meatballs into the pan in a single layer and cook for 3 minutes, or until browned.

5.When done, place all the meatballs in the pan, add cooked bell pepper mixture in it along with eggplant, stir in water and tomatoes and simmer for 30 minutes at low heat setting until thoroughly cooked.

6.Serve straight away.

Per serving: Calories: 265 kcal Total Fat: 18 g Saturated Fat: 0 g Cholesterol: 47 mg Sodium: 153 mg Total Carbs: 12 g Fiber: 4.6 g Protein: 17 g

Slow-Cooked Lemon Chicken

Prep time: 20 minutes

Cook time: 7 hours

Serves: 4

What you need:

- 1 teaspoon dried oregano
- ¼ teaspoon ground black pepper

- 2 tablespoons butter, unsalted
- 1-pound chicken breast, boneless, skinless
- ¼ cup chicken broth, low sodium
- ¼ cup water
- 1 tablespoon lemon juice
- 2 cloves garlic, minced
- 1 teaspoon fresh basil, chopped

Method:

1. Combine oregano and ground black pepper in a small bowl. Rub mixture on the chicken.

2. Melt the butter in a medium-sized skillet over medium heat. Brown the chicken in the melted butter and then transfer the chicken to the slow cooker.

3. Place chicken broth, water, lemon juice and garlic in the skillet. Bring it to a boil so it loosens the browned bits from the skillet. Pour over the chicken.

4. Cover, set slow cooker on high for 2½ hours or low for 5 hours.

5. Add basil and baste chicken. Cover, cook on high for an additional 15–30 minutes or until chicken is tender.

Per serving: Calories: 197 kcal Total Fat: 9 g Saturated Fat: 5 g Cholesterol: 99 mg Sodium: 57 mg Total Carbs: 1 g Fiber: 0.3 g Sugar: 0 g Protein: 26 g

Smothered Pork Chops and Sautéed Greens

Prep time: 20 minutes

Cook time: 60 minutes

Serves: 6

What you need:

- Smothered Pork Chops:
- 6 pork loin chops ("natural" center cut, bone-in)

- 1 tablespoon black pepper
- 2 teaspoons paprika
- 2 teaspoons granulated onion powder
- 2 teaspoons granulated garlic powder
- 1 cup and 2 tablespoons flour
- ½ cup canola oil
- 2 cups low-sodium beef stock
- 1 ½ cups fresh onions, sliced
- ½ cup fresh scallions, sliced on the bias
- Sautéed Greens:
- 8 cups fresh collard greens, chopped and blanched
- 2 tablespoons olive oil
- 1 tablespoon unsalted butter
- ¼ cup onions, finely diced
- 1 tablespoon fresh garlic, chopped
- 1 teaspoon crushed red pepper flakes
- 1 teaspoon black pepper
- 1 teaspoon vinegar (optional)

Method:

1. Preheat oven to 350° F.
2. Pork Chops:
3. Mix black pepper, paprika, onion powder and garlic powder together. Use half of mixture to season both sides of the pork chops and mix the other half with 1 cup flour.
4. Reserve 2 tablespoons of flour mix for later.
5. Lightly coat pork chops with seasoned flour.
6. Heat oil in large Dutch oven or oven-ready sauté pan (no rubber handles) on medium-high.

7.Fry pork chops for 2–4 minutes on each side or until desired crispness. Remove from pan and pour off all but 2 tablespoons of oil.

8.Cook onions until translucent, about 4–6 minutes. Stir in 2 tablespoons of reserved flour and mix well with onions for about 1 minute.

9.Slowly, add beef stock and stir until thickened.

10.Return pork chops to pan and coat with sauce. Cover or wrap with foil and cook in oven for at least 30–45 minutes at 350° F.

11.Remove from oven and let rest at least 5–10 minutes before serving.

12. Sautéed Greens:

13. To blanch greens, add greens to a pot of boiling water for 30 seconds.

14. Strain boiling water off and quickly transfer to ready bowl of ice and water.

15. Let cool, then strain and dry greens and set aside.

16. In large sauté pan on medium-high heat, melt butter and oil together. Add onions and garlic, cook until slightly browned, about 4–6 minutes.

17.Add collard greens and black and red pepper and cook for 5–8 minutes on high heat, stirring constantly.

18. Remove from heat; add vinegar if desired and stir.

Per serving: Calories: 464 kcal Total Fat: 28 g Saturated Fat: 5 g Cholesterol: 71 mg Sodium: 108 mg Total Carbs: 26 g Fiber: 1.3 g Sugar: 0 g Protein: 27 g

Pasta with Cheesy Meat Sauce

Prep time: 10 minutes

Cook time: 30 minutes

Serves: 6

What you need:

•½ box large-shaped pasta

•1-pound ground beef*

•½ cup onions, diced

•1 tablespoon onion flakes

•1½ cups beef stock, reduced or no sodium

•1 tablespoon Better Than Bouillon® beef, no salt added

•1 tablespoon tomato sauce, no salt added

•¾ cup Monterey or pepper jack cheese, shredded

•8 ounces cream cheese, softened

•½ teaspoon Italian seasoning

•½ teaspoon ground black pepper

•2 tablespoons French's® Worcestershire sauce, reduced sodium

Method:

1.Cook pasta noodles according to the directions on the box.

2.In a large sauté pan, cook ground beef, onions and onion flakes until the meat is browned.

3.Drain and add stock, bouillon and tomato sauce.

4.Bring to a simmer, stirring occasionally. Stir in cooked pasta, turn off heat, and add softened cream cheese, shredded cheese and seasonings (Italian seasoning, black pepper and Worcestershire sauce). Stir pasta mixture until cheese is melted throughout.

TIP: You can substitute ground turkey for beef.

Per serving: Calories: 502 kcal Total Fat: 30 g Saturated Fat: 14 g Cholesterol: 99 mg Sodium: 401 mg Total Carbs: 35 g Fiber: 1.7 g Sugar: 0 g Protein: 23 g

Aromatic Herbed Rice

Prep time: 10 minutes

Cook time: 15 minutes

Serves: 6

What you need:

- 2 tablespoons olive oil
- 3 cups cooked rice (don't overcook)
- 4–5 cloves fresh garlic, sliced thin
- 2 tablespoons fresh cilantro, chopped
- 2 tablespoons fresh oregano, chopped
- 2 tablespoons fresh chives, chopped
- ½ teaspoon red pepper flakes
- 1 teaspoon red wine vinegar

Method:

1. In a large sauté pan, heat olive oil on medium-high heat and lightly sauté garlic. Add rice, herbs and red pepper flakes and continue to cook for 2–4 minutes or until well-mixed.

2. Turn off heat, add vinegar, mix well and serve.

Per serving: Calories: 134 kcal Total Fat: 5 g Saturated Fat: 1 g Cholesterol: 0 mg Sodium: 6 mg Total Carbs: 21 g Fiber: 1.8 g Sugar: 0 g Protein: 2 g

Herb-Crusted Roast Leg of Lamb

Prep time: 10 minutes

Cook time: 45 minutes

Serves: 12

What you need:

- 1 4-pound leg of lamb

- 3 tablespoons lemon juice
- 1 tablespoon curry powder
- 2 cloves garlic, minced
- ½ teaspoon ground black pepper
- 1 cup onions, sliced
- ½ cup dry vermouth

Method:

1. Preheat oven to 400° F.

2. Place leg of lamb on a roasting pan. Sprinkle with 1 teaspoon of lemon juice.

3. Make paste with 2 teaspoons of lemon juice and the rest of the spices. Rub the paste onto the lamb.

4. Roast lamb in 400° F oven for 30 minutes.

5. Drain off fat and add vermouth and onions.

6. Reduce heat to 325° F and cook for an additional 1¾–2 hours. Baste leg of lamb frequently. When internal temperature is 145° F, remove from oven and let rest 3 minutes before serving.

Per serving: Calories: 292 kcal Total Fat: 20 g Saturated Fat: 9 g Cholesterol: 86 mg Sodium: 157 mg Total Carbs: 2 g Fiber: 0 g Sugar: 0 g Protein: 24 g

Baked Potatoes with Spicy Chickpea

Prep time: 10 minutes

Cook time: 10 minutes

Serves: 4-6

What you need:

- 4-6 baking potatoes, pricked all over
- Two tablespoons olive oil
- Two red onions, finely chopped

- Four cloves garlic, grated or crushed
- 2cm ginger, grated
- Two tablespoons turmeric
- ½ -2 teaspoons of chili flakes (depending on how hot you like things)
- Two tablespoons cumin seeds
- Splash of water
- Two into 400g tins chopped tomatoes
- Two tablespoons unsweetened cocoa powder (or cacao)
- Two into 400g tins chickpeas (or kidney beans if you prefer) including the chickpea water
- Two yellow peppers (or whatever color you prefer!), chopped into bite size pieces
- Salt and pepper to taste (optional)
- Side salad (optional)

Method:

1. Preheat the oven to 200C so you can make all the ingredients you need.

2. Put your baking potatoes in the oven when the oven is hot enough, and cook them for an hour or till they are cooked as you want them.

3. Put the olive oil and chopped red onion in a big broad saucepan once the potatoes are in the oven and cook gently with the lid until the onions are soft but not brown for 5 minutes.

4. Remove the lid and add the garlic, cumin, ginger and chili. Cook on low heat for another minute, and then you add the turmeric and a tiny sprinkle of water and cook for another minute, keeping in minute not to let the saucepan get too dry.

5. Add cocoa (or cacao) powder, chickpeas (including chickpea water) and yellow pepper in the tomatoes. Boil it and simmer for 45 minutes at low heat until the sauce is thick and greasy

(but don't let it burn!). Stew will be handled roughly at the same time as the potatoes.

6.At last, mix in the two tablespoons of parsley and some salt and pepper, if desired, and serve the stew over the baked potatoes, maybe with a small side salad.

Per serving: Cals -220 Fat -9g Chol -0 Carb -21g Fiber -6g Protein -5

Aromatic Chicken

Prep time: 15 minutes

Cook time: 15 minutes

Serves: 1

What you need:

For the salsa

•One large tomato

•One bird's eye chili, finely chopped

•1tbsp capers, finely chopped

•5g parsley, finely chopped

•Juice 1/2 lemon

•For the chicken

•120g skinless, boneless chicken breast

•2tsp ground turmeric

•Juice 1/2 lemon

•1tbsp extra virgin olive oil

•50g kale, chopped

•20g red onion, sliced

•1tsp fresh ginger, finely chopped

•50g buckwheat

Method:

1.Heat the oven at 220oC/200oC fan/gas level 7

2.Cut the tomato thinly to make the salsa and make sure you hold as much of the liquid as possible. Mix with the chili, capers, lemon juice and parsley.

3.Marinate the chicken breast for 5-10 minutes with 1tsp of turmeric, lemon juice and half of the butter.

4.Heat the frying pan ovenproof; add the marinated chicken and cook each side for a minute until golden, then move to the oven for 8-10 minutes or until cooked through. Remove and cover with tape, then leave for 5 minutes to rest.

5.Then you cook the Kale in a 5-minutesute steamer. In the remaining oil, fry the onion and ginger until soft but not white, then put the cooked Kale and fry for one more minute.

6.Cook the buckwheat with the remaining turmeric as directed, and then serve.

Per serving: Calories- 73 Fat- 2.7g Protein (with bone)- 0.44g Total Cholesterol - 66mg

Buckwheat Noodles with Chicken kale & Miso Dressing

Prep time: 15 minutes

Cook time: 15 minutes

Serves: 2

What you need:

For the noodles

•2-3 handfuls of kale leaves (removed from the stem and roughly cut)

•3-4 shiitake mushrooms, sliced

•150 g / 5 oz. buckwheat noodles (100% buckwheat, no wheat)

•One teaspoon coconut oil or ghee

- One medium free-range chicken breast, sliced or diced
- One brown onion, finely diced
- One long red chili, thinly sliced (seeds in or out depending on how hot you like it)
- Two large garlic cloves, finely diced
- 2-3 tablespoons Tamari sauce (gluten-free soy sauce)

For the miso dressing

- One tablespoon Tamari sauce
- 1½ tablespoon fresh organic miso
- One tablespoon extra-virgin olive oil
- One teaspoon sesame oil (optional)
- One tablespoon lemon or lime juice

Method:

1. Bring a medium water saucepan to boil. Add the kale and cook until slightly withered, for 1 minute. Remove and set aside, then put the water back to the boil. Add the soba noodles and cook (usually about 5 minutes) according to packaging instructions. Set aside and rinse under cold water.

2. Meanwhile, in a little ghee or coconut oil (about a teaspoon), pan fry the shiitake mushrooms for 2-3 minutes, until lightly browned on either side. Sprinkle with salt from the sea, and set aside.

3. Heat the coconut oil or ghee in the same frying pan over medium to high heat. Stir in onion and chili for 2-3 minutes, and then add pieces of chicken. Cook over medium heat for 5 minutes, stirring a few times, and then add the garlic, tamari sauce and some splash of water. Cook for another 2-3 minutes, often stirring until chicken is cooked through.

4. Finally, add the kale and soba noodles and warm up by stirring through the chicken.

5. In the end, mix the miso dressing and drizzle over the noodles to keep all the beneficial probiotics alive and active in the miso.

Per serving: Calories: 210 Total Fat: 13g Saturated Fat: 1g

Sirt Super Salad

Prep time: 10 minutes

Cook time: 10 minutes

Serves: 1

What you need:

•50g rocket

•50g chicory leaves

•100g smoked salmon slices

•80g avocado, peeled, stoned and sliced

•40g celery, sliced

•20g red onion, sliced

•15g walnuts, chopped

•One large Medjool date, pitted and chopped

•1tbsp extra virgin olive oil

•1tbsp capers

•Juice 1/2 lemon

•10g parsley, chopped

•10g lovage or celery leaves, chopped

Method:

1.Mix all the ingredients, and your salad is ready.

Per serving: Calories: 274

Kale, Edamame and Tofu curry

Prep time: 5 minutes

Cook time: 20 minutes

Serves: 2

What you need:

- 2 1/2 of your five-day SIRT,
- Warm the curry.
- Easy to keep it cool or freeze for another day.
- Ready in 45 minutes
- 1 tbsp. rapeseed oil
- One large onion, chopped
- Four cloves garlic, peeled and grated
- One large thumb (7cm) fresh ginger, peeled and grated
- One red chili, deseeded and thinly sliced
- 1/2 tsp ground turmeric
- 1/4 tsp cayenne pepper
- 1 tsp paprika
- 1/2 tsp ground cumin
- 1 tsp salt
- 250g dried red lentils
- 1-liter boiling water
- 50g frozen soya edamame beans
- 200g firm tofu, chopped into cubes
- Two tomatoes, roughly chopped
- Juice of 1 lime
- 200g kale leaves stalk removed and torn

Method:

1. Put the oil over low-medium heat in a heavy-bottom pan. Add the turmeric, cayenne, cumin, paprika, and oil. Remove and mix again, before adding the red lentils.

2. Pour in the boiling water and cook for 10 minutes until the curry has a thick' •porridge' consistency, then reduce the heat and cook for another 20-30 minutes.

3.Add soya beans, tofu, and tomatoes and continue to cook for another 5 minutes. Add the juice of lime and kale leaves and cook until the kale is tender.

Per serving: calories, 14.5 gm fat, 3.9 gm sat. fat, 22.8 gm carbs, 113 mg sodium, 92 mg cholesterol, 83 mg calcium, 5.2 gm protein

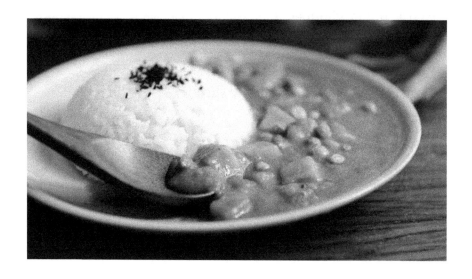

Lightning Source UK Ltd.
Milton Keynes UK
UKHW020818250521
384336UK00004B/91